Cultural and Ethnic Diversity

Cultural and Ethnic Diversity

A GUIDE FOR GENETICS PROFESSIONALS

Edited by Nancy L. Fisher, R.N., M.D., M.P.H.

Director, Medical Genetic Services, Seattle, Washington
Clinical Associate Professor of Pediatrics, University of Washington

The Johns Hopkins University Press
Baltimore and London

© 1996 The Johns Hopkins University Press
All rights reserved. Published 1996
Printed in the United States of America on acid-free paper
05 04 03 02 01 00 99 98 97 96   5 4 3 2 1

The Johns Hopkins University Press
2715 North Charles Street
Baltimore, Maryland 21218–4319
The Johns Hopkins Press Ltd., London

Library of Congress Cataloging-in-Publication Data will
be found at the end of this book.
A catalog record for this book is available from the British Library.

ISBN 0–8018–5346–x

Contents

Contributors

Kathleen Shaver Arnos, Ph.D., Director, Genetic Services, Gallaudet Research Institute, Gallaudet University, Washington, D.C.

Bruce A. Bernstein, Ph.D., Assistant Professor, Department of Pediatrics, and Adjunct Professor, Department of Anthropology, University of Connecticut, Storrs, Connecticut

Sechin Cho, M.D., Professor and Chair, Department of Pediatrics, University of Kansas School of Medicine, Wichita Genetic Services, Wichita, Kansas

Margaret Cunningham, R.N., Genetic Nurse, Genetic Services Center, Gallaudet University, Washington, D.C.

Clair A. Francomano, M.D., Chief, Medical Genetics Branch, National Center for Human Genome Research, National Institutes of Health, Bethesda, Maryland; and Associate Professor of Medicine and Pediatrics, Johns Hopkins University School of Medicine, Center for Medical Genetics, Johns Hopkins Hospital, Baltimore, Maryland

Mark A. Greenstein, M.D., Associate Professor of Pediatrics, Divisions of Developmental and Behavioral Pediatrics and Human Genetics, University of Connecticut School of Medicine, Farmington, Connecticut; and Associate Attending Staff, Saint Francis Hospital and Medical Center, Hartford, Connecticut

Lynn Hauck, M.A., M.S., Genetic Counselor, Section of Medical Genetics, Department of Pediatrics, University of Arizona Health Science Center, Tucson, Arizona

Jamie Israel, M.S., Genetic Counselor, Genetic Services Center, Gallaudet University, Washington, D.C.

Jack H. Jung, M.D., Professor and Chair, Division of Medical Genetics, and Director, Regional Medical Genetics Centre, Children's Hospital of Western Ontario, University of Western Ontario, London, Ontario

Ursula M. Knoki-Wilson, C.N.M., M.S.N., Supervisory Nurse Midwife, Fort Defiance Indian Hospital, Navajo Indian Health Service, Fort Defiance, Arizona

David C. Koehn, M.Sc., Genetic Counselor, Department of Medical Genetics, B.C. Children's Hospital, Vancouver, British Columbia

Lillian Lew, M.Ed., R.D., Director, Southeast Asian Health Project, St. Mary's Medical Center, Long Beach, California

Elena Lopez-Rangel, M.D., M.Sc., Fellow, Department of Pediatrics, Division of Biochemical Diseases, B.C. Children's Hospital, University of British Columbia, Vancouver, British Columbia

Kermit B. Nash, Ph.D., Professor, School of Social Work, University of North Carolina at Chapel Hill, and Principal Investigator, Psychosocial Research Division, Duke-UNC Comprehensive Sickle Cell Program, Chapel Hill, North Carolina

Shivanand R. Patil, Ph.D., Professor, Department of Pediatrics, and Director, Cytogenetics Laboratory, University of Iowa, Iowa City, Iowa

Rose Anne Pillay, B.Sc. B.Ed., Research Student, Department of Medical Genetics, B.C. Children's Hospital, Vancouver, British Columbia

Anne C. Spencer, M.S., Genetic Counselor, Perinatology, St. Luke's Regional Medical Center, Boise, Idaho

Marie D. Strazar, Ph.D., Director, History and Humanities Program, State Foundation on Culture and Arts, Honolulu, Hawaii

Joseph Telfair, Dr.P.H., M.S.W., M.P.H., Assistant Professor, School of Public Health, Maternal and Child Health, University of North Carolina at Chapel Hill, Chapel Hill, North Carolina

Helen Thumann, M.A., Reading Teacher, Transitional Department, Texas School for the Deaf, Austin, Texas

Foreword

The knowledge gained in the last few decades through molecular genetic techniques and the human genome projects has revolutionized the practice of medical genetics. However, the ways in which individuals and families will use that knowledge depend upon their own personal background and values. Health professionals providing genetic information and counseling will do a better job of communicating if they are aware of, and attuned to, the broad spectrum of approaches and backgrounds that individuals and families may bring to a counseling session. Some value systems can be expected to clash, some families may have a mixture of traditional and other types of values, but no family comes to genetic counseling without a serious problem for which they are seeking help.

Genetic counseling is defined as a communication process, a two-way experience in which both the counselor and the counselee provide information, listen, share, and, it is to be hoped, gain insights. Health professionals cannot help but come to a genetic counseling session with a cultural background of their own. Some individuals recognize the individual nature of their own values; others assume that everyone feels and thinks as they do. This book should help readers become aware of their own cultural background and inherent values as well as the diversity of other approaches that are part of the modern North American and world perspective. This book is a timely and valuable contribution.

There has been no previous comprehensive cultural source book for genetics professionals. Nancy Fisher has brought together an outstanding group of authors (expert because of their background, experience, and sensitivity) to discuss the issues that may be part of a genetic counseling session, and that may need to be discussed for families to be able to explore their options. What a marvelous diversity, and what an amazing spectrum! The reader is in for an adventure and an awakening! Probably at no time in history has so much been known about so many cultures. Nor have there ever been so many choices and options available, medically and socially, for an individual with a genetic problem. There is no simple right way! An individual, a family may choose what seems right for them and, we hope, will receive "person-appropriate" genetic care.

Every chapter in this book emphasizes the importance of respect in dealing with the individuals of a particular cultural or ethnic background. The authors have provided guidelines about nonverbal as well as verbal communication. Strong messages explain what could be considered unacceptable or rude behavior. Specific information (although, of course, generalizations) will help to alert genetics professionals to potentially sensitive areas. How fortunate we are to have this book become available just as the world is becoming smaller.

I found that I couldn't put the book down. I went from chapter to chapter, making comparisons, fascinated by the diversity. I know I will want to reread the good advice in each chapter before seeing an individual or a family from a specific ethnic or cultural group. No book is ever complete, and so there will be some additional group, some new information to be discussed in the future, and some descriptions of groups that will need to be expanded. Nevertheless, this is a grand beginning on a challenging and much-needed subject.

JUDITH G. HALL, M.D.
Professor and Head, Department of Pediatrics, B.C. Children's Hospital
Professor, Medical Genetics, University of British Columbia
Vancouver, British Columbia

Acknowledgments

The editor and chapter authors are indebted to many individuals for their support and enthusiasm in the writing of this book.

Let us first thank Wendy Harris for her wisdom, original concept, and editorial expertise; Miriam Tillman for her final text editing; and all the other staff members at the Johns Hopkins University Press who provided their time and talent to this process.

We express our deep appreciation to Ann Robertson and Ingrid Maksirisombat for their research skills. We also appreciate the helpful suggestions provided by Melanie Ito, M.D., Odette Sueda, M.D., Ann Robertson, M.L.S., Larry W. Larson, M.D., and Margo I. Van Allen, M.D.

Our heartfelt gratitude is also extended to all the typists in the various institutions, especially Cheri Dawson, Nichole Stromberg, and Sarah Farley.

Last, we are especially indebted to our patients and colleagues who so generously entrusted us with information about their cultures so that we may all begin to understand our pluralistic society.

Introduction

We live in an era of diversity. Very few cultures or countries are homogeneous. Wars as well as advances in communication, transportation, engineering, and computer technology have brought the peoples of the world closer together. In previous decades, individuals lived close to others of similar beliefs and habits, which often led to ethnocentric behavior: the belief that one's own culture is superior and contains rules of the correct way—perhaps even the only way—to think and behave. In fact, this behavior helped to bind people together and gave order to society. Humankind learned that interactions were easier with individuals who were similar, and tended to avoid those individuals perceived as different.

This book begins to address those differences in order to assist medical genetics professionals (physicians, geneticists, and genetics counselors) to better communicate with their patients. Because words written on paper are biased by the opinion and experiences of the authors, it is impossible to write an unbiased chapter about culture. To help minimize bias, authors who represent a specific cultural or ethnic group were chosen to write about their own culture and heritage. If this was not possible, an individual who had lived in or was very familiar with a given culture wrote the chapter. The book is not comprehensive, since not every culture is represented, but no culture was purposely omitted; rather, the chapters provide a sampling of cultural diversity.

To write about behavior, one usually has to delineate groups. This does not mean that everyone in a particular group, society, or culture thinks or behaves the same way. Such classifications are often arbitrary, serving as general indications that some, many, or even most people of that group may hold specific beliefs.

Each chapter contains information on historical and geographical background, cultural influences (religion, family traditions, modes of communication, beliefs about health), implications for genetic services, a brief summary, and bibliographic references. The summary not only reinforces the major concepts in the chapter but also affords the reader a quick reference in times of "emergency."

CULTURE

Culture is not limited to specific racial groups, geographical areas, spoken language, religious beliefs, dress, sexual orientation, or socioeconomic status. It is too complex. Culture consists of the shared patterns, knowledge, meaning, and behaviors of a social group. Most people cannot define their own culture because they take so much for granted. Culture seems to be something someone *else* possesses.

It should be remembered that without differences, life could be awfully boring. Even the fast-food restaurants dotting the United States attest to variety: fish and chips, tacos, burgers, pizza. American food is as varied as the terrain. Just as individuals learn to enjoy different foods, they can learn to understand and embrace other differences. No single culture has all the answers.

In the study of cultural and human diversity, the deeper one delves, the more similarities one uncovers. Individuals want to live, learn, have meaningful relationships, and count in society. How they achieve these goals is largely defined by their culture, which may have been affected by geographical area, the whims of nature, the development of society, and access to water, food, and other necessities.

Western technological development has not always improved society and the health of its members. The widespread use of refined sugars brought dental caries. Industrialization disrupted community life and polluted the land, air, and water. This progress manifests itself in a long list of health problems, from asthma to cancer. The drive toward materialistic success has increased the incidence of ulcers, hypertension, heart attacks, and other stress-related diseases. To some groups, like the Amish, it seems reasonable to distance oneself from such a culture. This distance between cultures may bring safety but may also create barriers to communication and genetic evaluation.

Cultural relativism, learning about another belief system, includes respectful behavior and communication between groups of people—in this case, between patients and their genetics professionals. New immigrants face stresses and strains that are economic and may have been discriminatory. Many individuals may be hesitant about or may fear the counseling session. A polite and patient counselor can minimize this fear.

It is hoped that information in this book will give the practitioner some awareness that because of experience, race, socioeconomic status, sex, religious beliefs, sexual orientation, education, or health status, individuals may have different customs and beliefs that need to be respected. Without this understanding, genetic counseling and evaluation cannot approach being nondirective, let alone appropriate to the patient.

Western medicine itself is a culture arising from a set of shared beliefs about the nature of reality and disease. These include a belief in science and the beneficial results of technology: a belief that the mysteries of nature are ultimately knowable; a belief that the body, like a machine, can be taken apart and "fixed" when it is not working properly. Such beliefs, unique to Western medicine, contrast sharply with belief systems of many traditional societies and ethnic groups, which have their unique views. As a culture, Western medicine has its own "language," standards of care, and body of knowledge.

Human genetics can be defined as a subculture of Western medicine. There is a specific language (DNA fingerprinting, Southern blots, hemizygosity, etc.). The patterns of behavior are sometimes different from those of Western medicine: not only is the patient evaluated and counseled but genetics professionals also actively seek out family members at risk. Additionally, genetic researchers are driven in their desire to map the human genome, relieve suffering from genetic disease, and help humankind. However, the definition of genetic burden may vary from culture to culture, even from the researcher to the clinician.

As researchers strive for the goals that they see as worthy, genetic counselors should be aware that their own basic premises about the nature of reality—for example, that scientific knowledge is good and useful, that humans should try to know whatever can be known about themselves, that manipulation of the building blocks of life for human "betterment" is desirable—may not be shared by members of other cultural groups. Some religious groups see probing and manipulation of genes as "playing God" or interfering with fate, and insist that because the genetically handicapped have their appointed role to play in life, they should not be screened out of existence. The Human Genome Project itself is running up against stiff resistance from a number of indigenous groups (Native Americans to Australian aborigines) who fear that their genes, viewed by the Human Genome Project as a valuable part of human "diversity," will be harvested and utilized by scientists to improve the genetic strength of the very groups who have been oppressing these indigenous groups for hundreds of years.

The scientific drive to understand human genes has led to a revolution in information. The development and application of the new genetic technologies is only in its infancy. This knowledge is exciting and awe inspiring, yet at the same time bewildering and frightening. New gene discoveries prompt new questions every day. How do we disseminate that knowledge? Even as genetic counselors give updated information about prenatal testing, and geneticists evaluate, diagnose, and test DNA when applicable, is there time to think about the impact of the information on the patient?

Genetic counseling is provided by individuals, not robots. A robot would have no compassion, no past experiences, no good or bad feelings about patients. Robots could give nonjudgmental, nondirective counseling—"just the facts!" Patients then could make informed decisions, uninfluenced by the "personal baggage" of the counselor. Many genetic counselors believe they, too, can provide nonjudgmental counseling, but even simply using language to talk about "the facts" conveys implicit assumptions and directions—it is not nondirective. On the other hand, genetics is very *personal.* The decisions to be made can be extremely difficult and have far-reaching consequences. Needless to say, humans need compassion, insight, and empathy to deliver this information. The impact of this newfound knowledge is complex and includes the values and education of the counselor, the culture and beliefs of the patient, the gender of the counselor and the patient, and the new knowledge itself.

GENETICS AND CULTURE

Each genetic counselor is part of a culture, evident in dress, cuisine, religion, norms of life, family size, and age. All counselors have past experiences that influence their interaction with others. Their education teaches that one purpose of genetics is to help those with genetic diagnoses reach their full potential. For these and other reasons, genetic counselors believe that patients should be educated regarding appropriate tests, the risk of genetic disorders, and other critical issues.

Patients have choices. But what verbal or nonverbal cues does the counselor give the patient if the answer is "incorrect"—that is, not in agreement with the answer the counselor expects or desires? In many such instances, when the counselor and the patient do not share the same culture or beliefs, the counselor sometimes repeats the information, believing that the information was not clear or the patient did not understand. However, it is the counselor who did not understand. The anxiety and difficulty of decision-making can only be increased in such instances.

Physicians, too, can cause anxiety in their relationships with patients (Kleinman, 1979). After all, the medical encounter, including an examination of the semi-nude or naked body, is very personal. Medical assessment may involve not only examining the body but also entering the realm of a person's essence, DNA; inquiring about very personal family issues; and revealing imperfections—"bad" genes.

"Perfect" individuals living in what they perceive to be a perfect society may not want to hear or learn about imperfections. In fact, genetics as a whole may be in conflict with many cultural beliefs, including Western beliefs. Other individuals may view this information as a "bad mark" against their family, including their ancestors. The beliefs about hope for the future, fate, individualism, materialism, spiritualism, time, directness, family, and honesty have a powerful impact on decision-making.

Consider, for example, the individual who is informed that he has the gene for

Huntington disease. For some, values are shaken to the core. In this instance, science has declared that fate exists: the patient will develop Huntington disease. Mastery over nature is an illusion; time no longer dominates but is limited; future orientation is dissolved; materialism offers no comfort. Why accumulate things for a future that no longer exists? Genetics and this individual's societal values have clashed. However, every person will handle the information differently. Another individual who believes in fate and reincarnation may truly be calm and accepting of the information. This may help explain why not everyone is clamoring for genetic tests.

In another case, a person diagnosed as a carrier of cystic fibrosis or sickle cell disease is informed that her relatives should be notified. But she may not have spoken with the individuals in question for years. Perhaps this person is considered "not part of the family." Suddenly, individual choice and privacy are challenged. She is reminded that someone with whom she has no personal bond has "essence" or genetic material in common with her. Moreover, she is informed she has a *responsibility* toward that person. No wonder some patients become angry or use denial as a mechanism to protect themselves and preserve their value systems.

Not all choices and cultural differences should be reduced to individual defensiveness. People do and can say no. Choice should be real, not an illusion of control. People make different choices for different reasons. A couple with a twenty-year infertility problem may decline amniocentesis or chorionic villus sampling, seeing the potential loss of their fetus as a greater burden than other outcomes. Other couples may see abortion as a way to prevent future suffering to the unborn fetus, as a selfish act, or as immoral. These different beliefs and values should be respected, not resented.

It could be argued that health care providers already practice cross-cultural medicine, since they see patients who are not of the Western medical or genetic culture. This culture has its unique traits, which result from special training or status. For example, genetics has its own language. An "uneventful" pregnancy for the geneticist is very eventful for the couple. A "positive" family history is usually very negative for the patient (R. Rapp, personal communication, 1994). The authors of this book wish to go a step further in dealing with diversity. We want readers to examine carefully their own stereotypes.

RACE AND CULTURE

Race does not always define culture, nor does religion, nor does residence. Is the fourth-generation Swedish American more "American" than the tenth-generation African American in the United States? If both come from educated families and attended liberal arts colleges, they probably share more culturally than most suspect. Just because two people have blond hair and blue eyes does not make their cultures the same. Stereotypes may have accuracy of description, but they run the risk of distortion through a lack of understanding. It is normal to laugh at oneself; it is not acceptable to explicitly ridicule others. Overweight people may tell "fat" jokes, but it is offensive for thin people to tell the same jokes.

If there is cultural diversity in a supposedly homogeneous society, difficulties multiply when individuals have a different first language, come from a different geographical area, have different expectations of physicians, or have an education rooted in spiritualism rather than science. Their beliefs and values are not wrong; they are just different. Neither is better nor worse, just distinctive. Those of us involved in Western medicine must remember that we all too quickly label as "wrong" those whose world is not science based.

COMMUNICATION

Medicine, including genetics, is not only a science but also a process of communication. A researcher can design the best case-control study and have wonderful financial backing, but if the individual or group approached perceives the researcher to be rude, no information—or misinformation—will be conveyed.

Health care providers must pay careful attention to what is said and heard. Even when two people speak the same language, communication can be difficult. For example, a young woman with Marfan syndrome was cautioned, because of her mildly dilated aorta, to consider not having children. She (mis)heard that she *could* not have children, and thought she was infertile due to Marfan syndrome. She stopped using contraception and became pregnant.

What is said and how it is interpreted are important. There is a difference between "should not" and "could not," or being told one has the *gene* for a specific disorder and having the disease itself. Providers must pay close attention to patients' responses because that information can change how individuals view themselves, develop or maintain relationships with others, sustain earning power, and form other perceptions of life. These issues are even more important in a cross-cultural setting, where communication may be more difficult. Additionally, stigmatization, self-esteem, and other traits may be affected by decision-making that the counselor does not understand.

An interaction involves at least two people. Both have their own beliefs, values, and behaviors. When these are similar, the interaction usually flows smoothly. Similar speech patterns, gestures, outward appearance, and dress make one feel comfortable. However, if the speech rhythm or pronunciation is altered or the dress too different, either individual may feel uncomfortable and develop a variety of defense mechanisms. People may not answer when addressed or may answer yes to everything, regardless of their true feelings. Some may just leave the situation entirely, either physically or mentally. Others become authoritative or critical.

Table I.1. Suggestions for Selecting an Interpreter

- Choose an individual trained in medical terminology.
- If such an individual is not available, select someone who is not a member of the patient's family to avoid family biases or influences.
- Choose an interpreter of the same sex as the patient, of comparable age, or older than the patient. Information about sensitive or intimate topics is more readily given to such people. Older individuals signify authority and trust.
- Talk with the interpreter beforehand to establish an approach.
- Have a quiet, unhurried approach. Take time to seat everyone. Learn to use a few key introductory words in the patient's language.
- When speaking or listening, watch the patient and not the interpreter. Use short, simple statements.
- Address the patient in the second person (i.e., "you"). Ask how the patient wishes to be addressed.
- Do not expect word-for-word translation.
- Expect long conversations between the patient and interpreter, but do not accept "no" and "yes" for responses at the conclusion of them. Ask for substantial interpretation.
- Ask the interpreter what the patient's expectations, fears, and concerns are.
- If the interpreter speaks several languages, inquire of the interpreter whether the patient may hold any animosity for the ethnic group the interpreter may be viewed as representing.

Difference breeds discomfort, and everyone wants to feel comfortable. This book is intended to help the reader feel more comfortable with these differences in a clinical setting.

In most situations, it is not possible to ethnically match a counselor and a patient for each minority group. Languages are highly distinctive, having different nuances and idioms. Even when the genetic counselor is familiar with the patient's first language, an interpreter may be essential in the counseling session to help with medical meanings.

The use of interpreters carries distinct limitations and drawbacks. Translation adds time to the counseling session. Interpreters may censor or translate information into what they think the practitioner wants to hear. Additionally, they may be embarrassed to translate some of the information presented. As the counselor's communication style affects the encounter, so does the interpreter's.

An individual of similar background is the best choice for an interpreter, with consideration given to socioeconomic status and class. The patient's permission should be obtained before asking someone from the waiting room to serve as an interpreter; otherwise, it may be viewed as an invasion of privacy. Table I.1 gives suggestions for selecting an interpreter.

Table I.2. Questions to Include in Taking a Patient's History

- What do you think caused the problem?
- What kind of treatment should you receive?
- What are the most important results you hope to receive from the treatment or counseling?
- What do you fear the most about this information?
- How will this information alter your life?
- What would you like from me, the counselor?
- How has this condition altered your life?
- What are your worries relative to this condition?
- Will this condition, if it occurs, present problems in your community or family?
- Who makes decisions about matters of importance in the family?
- What is your social support system?

Source: Adapted from Kleinman (1979)

Counselors may lessen the distance between the patient and themselves through respect and appropriate communication. Kleinman (1979) suggests appropriate questions for the patient history-taking, which can be modified and utilized in genetics, as shown in table I.2. Counselors should facilitate the decision-making by families, if culturally appropriate, by doing two-step prenatal counseling: first, expressing an interest in the patient's thoughts, and second, if necessary, compromising, remembering that the concept of burden varies. If the world was populated primarily by Einsteins, individuals with an IQ of 130 would be considered intellectually challenged. If a society is based on farming, the impact of a lower IQ may not be as great as that of a limb-reduction deficit.

SUMMARY

This book is intended as the first step in helping those in genetics provide more effective service to people in diverse communities. From 1980 to 1990 in the United States, the white population increased 9.8 percent, the Hispanic population increased 53.0 percent, and the Asian–Pacific Islander population increased 100.0 percent. Whereas one in four people in the world is Chinese, one in four people in the United States is Hispanic or nonwhite. It is only a matter of time before geneticists or genetic counselors will encounter patients from a culture different from their own. Hopefully, along the way, counselors will clarify their beliefs and will glean some useful information about the beliefs and customs of their diverse clientele.

Ultimately, this book is intended to facilitate acknowledgment of and respect for different cultural heritages. After all, without diversity—both genetic and cultural—our species will not survive.

REFERENCES

Brodsky, C. M. 1983. Culture and disability behavior. *Western Journal of Medicine* 139:892–99.

Clark, M. M. 1983. Cultural context of medical practice. *Western Journal of Medicine* 139:806–10.

Fisher, N. L. 1992. Ethnocultural approaches to genetics. *Pediatric Clinics of North America* 39:55–64.

Haffner, L. 1992. Translation is not enough: Interpreting in a medical setting. *Western Journal of Medicine* 157:255–59.

Kleinman, A. 1979. *Patients and Healers in the Context of Culture: An Exploration of the Borderland between Anthropology, Medicine, and Psychiatry.* Berkeley: University of California Press.

Lazarus, E. S. 1990. Falling through the cracks: Contradictions and barriers to care in a prenatal clinic. *Medical Anthropology* 12:269–87.

Marston, D. 1992. The challenge of cross-cultural medicine. *Physicians Management* 1:18–25.

Ralhman, B. K. 1988. Reproductive technology and the commodification of life. In Baruch, F. H., and D'Adamo, A. F. (eds.), *Embryos, Ethics, and Women's Rights: Exploring the New Reproductive Technologies.* New York: Harrington Park Press.

Randall-David, E. 1989. Strategies for working with culturally diverse communities and clients. U.S. Department of Health and Human Resources. MCH no. 11373. Washington, D.C.: GPO.

Rapp, R. 1988. Chromosomes and communication: The discourse of genetic counseling. *Medical Anthropolgy Quarterly* 2:143–55.

———. 1990. *Constructing Amniocentesis in Uncertain Terms: Negotiating Gender in American Culture,* pp. 28–42. Boston: Beacon Press.

Rothenberg, K. H., and Thomson, E. J. (eds.). 1994. *Women and Prenatal Testing.* Columbus: Ohio State University Press.

Scheper-Hughes, N. 1990. Difference and danger: The cultural dynamics of childhood stigma, rejection, and rescue. *Cleft Palate Journal* 27:301–10.

Strauss, R. P. 1990. Culture, health care, and birth defects in the United States: An introduction. *Cleft Palate Journal* 27:275–78.

U.S. Bureau of the Census, Public Information Office. 1991. Patient population distribution for United States by race and Hispanic origin, 1980 and 1990. Washington, D.C.: GPO.

Cultural and Ethnic Diversity

·

1

European Culture in North America

Anne C. Spencer, M.S.

The majority of North Americans are of European ancestry. As a result, many Americans' beliefs, customs, and traditions resemble those of their European relatives. Still, these Americans are not simply carbon copies of Europeans; for a variety of reasons, many aspects of American culture are distinctive. History can provide insight into American culture and how it differs from others.

HISTORY AND GEOGRAPHY

On the whole, the Europeans who originally came to North America chose to leave their homelands for specific reasons. Traveling across the Atlantic Ocean was a major undertaking, and people did not usually make such a decision lightly. In general, therefore, there is a selection bias between the people who stayed in Europe and the people who traveled to the New World. These latter individuals had to be strongly motivated, willing to take initiative and accept great risk in return for a chance at a better life.

The explorers (from the British Isles, Spain, Portugal, France, Holland, and Italy) arrived first, seeking adventure and profit. Then came settlers (primarily from these same countries), escaping from religious or political persecution and hoping for economic opportunities. To succeed in the New World, these people needed to fight disease, famine, and drought, and clashes with Native Americans (Hanson, 1992). The characteristics associated with the original explorers and settlers are in many ways the hallmarks of American culture: individualism, entrepreneurial spirit, industriousness, practicality, ambition, and a desire for religious and ideological freedom.

Throughout U.S. history, Europeans have continued to immigrate to the United States. By the nineteenth and twentieth centuries, immigrants had arrived from all over Europe—the British Isles, Germany, Scandinavia, Russia, Italy, Eastern Europe, and the Mediterranean. While much of North American culture derives from its European roots, there have been other influences as well.

From the beginning, Europeans interacted with Native Americans. And while European diseases and aggression eventually decimated the native population, the early and continuing interaction with Native Americans certainly affected the newly developing American culture. Another non-European group present in America's infancy—the African slaves—were brought to do much of the hard labor necessary to clear and farm the land. Later, groups of Chinese immigrants served as cheap labor, building railroads necessary for westward migration.

All these groups—European and non-European—both adapted to their new country and retained practices of their own. The result, often referred to as a "melting pot," comprises people from many different backgrounds absorbed into a common but constantly changing society. While this term inaccurately suggests a goal of cultural homogeneity, it successfully conveys that each group coming to the United States contributes to the cuisine, arts, music, literature, folkways, and ultimately the culture of the country (Hanson, 1992).

The geography of the land also contributed to its culture. The varied landscape allowed a variety of subcultures to develop in different regions of the country. Thus, there is the industry of the Northeast, the plantations of the South, ranching in the West, and fishing and shipping along the coasts, lakes, and rivers. The vastness of the United States also allowed many settlers to have their own pieces of land. Americans of European ancestry have always enjoyed the privacy and freedom that comes with having a space of their own. However, the size of the country also made it difficult for people to travel and communicate with family, friends, government, and business associates. To combat these problems, Americans developed a number of systems for traveling across distances quickly (railroads, highways, and air travel) and for communicating cross-country (telegraphs, telephones, radios, and televisions). Partially because of the geography of the country, Americans have become dependent on their mobility and their technology.

All these factors—the personality and values of the settlers, the mixing of European and non-European cultures, and the expanse and geographic variation of the North American continent itself—contributed to create a unique American dominant culture, quite distinct from its primarily European roots. Because of its pluralistic beginnings, this culture values freedom, privacy, and diversity, which complicates generalizing about Americans of European descent. Still, these values are themselves unifying.

RELIGION

Given that an important motivating factor of early immigration was escape from religious persecution, it is not surprising that the First Amendment of the U.S. Constitution protects freedom of religion. Like the bulk of their ancestors, most Americans of European descent are Christian; Christianity influences a variety of public and private institutions: businesses are more likely to be closed on Sunday than on any other day of the week; baccalaureate services are held in conjunction with public and private school graduations; Christmas is a national holiday; and political officials and trial witnesses swear on the Bible. However, the fact that most Americans call themselves Christian in no way means that they share identical (or even similar) religious beliefs and practices. Of the 86.5 percent of Americans who espouse Christianity, 26 percent are Roman Catholic, 19 percent are Baptist, 8 percent are Methodist, 5 percent are Lutheran (*San Jose Mercury News,* 10 April 1991), and the remainder belong to hundreds of smaller denominations (Mead, 1990). Of the people who claim to be affiliated with a religion, many do not practice their stated beliefs. And a number of Americans of European descent are actively agnostic or atheistic. Because beliefs about family structure, reproductive technology, contraception, health care, abortion, and death and funeral rituals vary greatly with religious beliefs, it is important for health care providers to ascertain their patients' specific beliefs rather than assume values based on ethnicity or stated religious affiliation.

On the whole Americans of European ancestry do not consider themselves superstitious. However, many individuals may engage in some superstitious behavior. For example, they may believe the number thirteen, walking under ladders, spilling salt, and breaking a mirror can cause bad luck. They may also knock on wood to ward off misfortune. Even when behavior is motivated by superstitions, people would probably say that they don't believe that their actions will actually have any impact on the course of events.

FAMILY

Americans of European descent consider the traditional family to consist of a mother (who raises the children and takes care of household tasks), a father (who works outside the home and heads the family), and their biological children. The number of children varies considerably from family to family. Many couples have only one or two children, and with so few offspring they are heavily invested in these children being healthy, intelligent, and surviving to adulthood. Extended family is more likely to be seen as "relatives" than "family," and does not play a major role in child-rearing or family decision-making (Hanson, 1992). While most Americans of European descent still think of this as a typical family structure, the increasing number of women entering the work force, a high divorce rate, and increasing out-of-wedlock births, as well as a growing acceptance of homosexual couples raising children, have all resulted in a high percentage of families not fitting the traditional family model.

Single-parent households (often headed by women) are increasingly common, as are families in which both parents work outside the home. In both cases, children often spend large parts of their day with other relatives or in daycare centers, where paid child-care professionals look after the children. These trends also result in families in which both parenting and money-earning tasks are more equally shared between adults in the household. However, child-rearing still tends to be more the mother's responsibility. It is common for only one parent, generally the mother, to accompany a child to a doctor's appointment.

As parents marry or remarry, many children end up with step-parents, half-siblings, and step-siblings. These "blended families" pose a challenge to someone taking a family history, and it is important to clarify biological relationships between individuals in the family tree. "Blended" families may also increase the tension within households.

Marriage generally occurs between unrelated individuals; however, children can result from consanguineous relationships. This generally happens in the context of cousin marriage or from an incestuous rape. In the former situation, one can usually obtain this information by asking the parents if they are blood relatives. In the case of incestuous rape, it is often more difficult to elicit such a history, as the mother is usually young and either too afraid or too embarrassed to disclose this information. Because consanguineous mating is not socially acceptable, one should be tactful in discussing the possibility with an individual or family.

Like consanguinity, false paternity can produce a socially awkward situation for the person (often a health care professional) who suspects it. In a medical setting, it is often considered best to discuss this concern privately with the mother and to develop a plan about who should know of the actual paternity.

Because family structures vary so greatly, it is important for a genetics professional not to make assumptions about the family, and to ask questions until information is clear. In most situations, families will not be offended by this questioning (although it may represent a breach of privacy), as they see its importance for the provision of medical services.

COMMUNICATION

The early British influence established English as the primary language and it has remained so despite the many waves of non-English-speaking immigrants. American accents differ from British, Australian, and Canadian accents. Accents and dialects vary within the country as well, and there are some areas of the country in which Spanish is commonly spoken. However, these are the exceptions, and it is generally expected that Americans of European ancestry will be able to communicate through written and spoken standard American English.

Americans of European descent have also developed nonverbal, or body, language. It is generally accepted that two people will stand about arm's distance apart for ordinary communication. This is close enough to easily be heard, but not so close as to jeopardize people's feelings of privacy. Touching (with the exception of handshakes) is generally reserved for intimate relationships of friends and family. Typically, when two people are introduced to each other they will shake right hands (never left hands). A firm handshake is considered a sign of a strong person. Good eye contact indicates strength and honesty. A person who avoids eye contact may be considered "shifty" or untrustworthy. A variety of hand and body gestures carry important meaning, but also vary greatly with region, subculture, or the age of the person using the gesture.

CULTURE

The values that Americans of European descent share are, in many ways, the values that brought their ancestors to America and the values that allowed them to succeed in the rugged New World.

Productivity

On the whole, Americans of European ancestry value productivity and prefer action over inaction. This value is exemplified by the common expression, "Don't just stand there, do something!" It also comes out more subtly in the way that they identify themselves and one another by their profession—what they do for a living—rather than by other aspects of their lives, such as who their parents are or where they live. As a result of valuing productivity, Americans of European ancestry tend to schedule very active days with little time for relaxation. If they do schedule time for relaxation they justify it, calling it "re-creation," to prepare them to work hard the next day. Even this leisure time is generally carefully planned.

Related to their value on productivity is a desire for practicality. In making important decisions, they generally give the practical consideration highest priority (over esthetic or emotional considerations). This orientation has led Americans to contribute more inventions to the world than any other citizens in human history (Kohls, 1989). Americans of European descent like to feel that they are working efficiently and tend to replace their old stuff with the newest time-saving gadget. Because of this pragmatism, they emphasize the rational side of their selves over the subjective and emotional.

In parts of the United States, emotions, which are seen as something that interferes with productivity and progress, must be put aside to behave in a logical, rational, and objective manner. When Americans of European descent do choose the esthetic or emotional over the practical, they may feel apologetic or embarrassed by such "indulgence." It is common for a parent whose child has received a severe diagnosis to apologize for crying. This is not to imply that they don't allow themselves feelings, only that they must constantly find the balance between practicality and emotions; it is often more socially acceptable to choose practicality.

These beliefs about productivity and practicality do not leave much room for ideas that occur in other cultures and some subcultures of American society: that work can be play, that inactivity can be productive, and that some of what Americans of European descent classify as labor serves little or no worthwhile purpose (Lakoff and Johnson, 1980, p. 67).

Time

The desire to be productive also makes Americans of European descent time conscious. They tend to structure and schedule their days, allowing them to get more accomplished. They often choose getting things done or being on time over their interpersonal relationships, cutting off discussions with friends, family, and coworkers rather than being late for an appointment or falling behind on a project.

Americans of European ancestry are generally aware of the time—not just what time it is but how much time they have (or do not have) for a given task. This awareness of time is aided by the fact that most Americans of European descent wear wristwatches. In fact, they are thrown off their schedules by people who do not share the same time "anxiety," and resent people who keep them waiting or who make them late for another appointment.

Americans of European descent view time as a precious limited commodity, which they treat in much the same way as they treat money (Lakoff and Johnson, 1980, pp. 7–9). Think of some of the phrases commonly used to refer to time: "You are *wasting* my time"; "How are you *spending* your time?"; "I've *invested* a lot of time in the project"; "He's living on *borrowed* time"; "You need to *budget* your time more wisely"; and "That ploy really *bought* us some time." The cultural metaphor that "time is money" probably grows from an industrialized society in which people are paid by the hour and are charged for services, such as telephone calls, based on the amount of time they use that service. Because time is perceived as such a precious commodity, it should be spent wisely and not squandered.

Individualism and Privacy

Individualism is perhaps the trait that most distinguishes Americans of European descent. Each person is expected to make his or her own decisions. People are seen as autonomous individuals whose behavior is aimed at personal goals. This belief about the importance of the individual has a strong effect on family structure, because the dependent nature of the child requires parents to postpone personal goals to take care of their child. Americans have pared down the number of people for whom they are responsible to the bare minimum (i.e., children under the age of eighteen). They believe that if parents raise their children successfully, the children will become increasingly self-reliant and eventually become independent from their parents; Americans of Euopean descent expect parents and adult children to live essentially independent lives. According to Caudill (1976) a three-month-old American infant learns to take care of and express its own needs to a much greater degree than a similarly aged Japanese infant. An elderly person may resent living with relatives as much as an adult child would resent having to move in with parents, because in both instances this indicates lost independence (Wong and Banerian, 1980).

Extended family does not generally play a role in the decision-making of Americans of European descent. They view choosing a marriage partner as a personal decision rather than a social contract between two families (Wong and Banerian, 1980). In this pared-down version of the family, government, rather than relatives, assumes responsibility for people in need by offering programs such as Social Security, welfare, and food stamps.

None of this is to imply that Americans of European ancestry do not love and care for their relatives. Instead, their ideal is to have a family in which people interact as equals. By requesting help or borrowing money from a relative, a person is admitting that he or she is not equal to the person from whom he or she is requesting help. Owing a person money or a favor gives the lender power over the borrower and makes equality impossible.

Preferences of the individual may come before those of the family or society, except in cases where such personal preferences interfere with others' freedoms. Much of modern psychological therapy in the United States is based on teaching individuals who they are and what they want, rather than on having them take responsibility for or change others' actions.

Individualism leads to privacy, which is also valued (Kohls, 1989). Single-occupant offices, private hospital rooms, and "a few moments all to myself" are desired by most in this society. Even in interactions with other people, a number of topics are too personal for public discussion: income, age, weight, cost of items, and childbearing plans.

Initiative and Responsibility

Americans of European ancestry value initiative and admire people who climb the ladder of success. Their cultural heroes are people like Abraham Lincoln, who was born in a log cabin, studied by a kerosene lamp, and, through hard work and determination, became president of the United

States. Conversely, European-Americans tend to have little respect for people who are fatalistic, seeing them as lazy, superstitious, or lacking initiative. The problems in these people's lives are presumed to result from their unwillingness to take responsibility for pursuing a better life (Kohls, 1989). In bookstores, shelves are often crammed with self-help books, which are intended to teach their readers how to improve their lives without help from others.

Belief that each person has control over his or her environment has led to the expectation that people should take credit only for what they accomplish individually. Alexis de Tocqueville observed this tendency in Americans in the 1830s: persons in a democracy "owe nothing to any man, they expect nothing from any man; they acquire the habit of always considering themselves as standing alone, and they are apt to imagine that their whole destiny is in their own hands" (p. 508). Looking outside of oneself for help, whether to a diety, fate, or another human being (even a relative), is perceived as a sign of weakness and lack of internal resourcefulness. While in many cultures it would be an embarrassment not to provide a job to a friend or relative, Americans of European descent tend to have negative feelings about nepotism.

Because of the belief that humans, not fate, control the environment, they work hard to create a better future, setting short- and long-term goals and developing programs to guarantee that they meet these goals. In fact, Americans are so recognized as planners that they are often invited by other countries to help plan and set goals (Kohls, 1989).

Equality

At the core of the view that individuals, rather than fate, are responsible for their own status and success or failure is the belief that "all men are created equal." Everyone, according to popular belief, has equal opportunity to succeed and anyone can grow up to be president (though history shows that many opportunities are, in reality, limited). The idea that people are to be judged on their own merits rather than which family they were born into or even what job they are doing, permeates much of social interaction.

This sense of egalitarianism precludes feeling one person is subordinate merely because she or he is performing a service (e.g., waiter, taxi driver, cashier), or because she or he is working for another individual. Americans of European ancestry feel very comfortable with a boss chatting and joking with employees. In fact, they are put off by a boss who is "bossy."

Egalitarianism is not limited to professional life. As discussed earlier,

Americans of European descent believe adult relatives should have an egalitarian relationship. The training of children to grow up to be equals begins early, and children are encouraged to challenge and question their teachers as evidence of independent thinking (Wong and Banerian, 1980). More and more children are growing up calling their teachers by their first names. Unlike many cultures, which encourage their children to imitate and respect elderly people, Americans of European descent encourage their children to grow up and surpass the achievements of their elders.

Affluence and Acquisitiveness

Compared to people in many other parts of the world, Americans of European descent are rich and can afford many things. They are likely to throw away items that are still potentially useful and that less affluent cultures might consider quite valuable. What they acquire is viewed as the natural benefit of their hard work. The corollary to this is that people who have less are viewed as not having worked as hard, and therefore do not deserve material benefits.

In their acquisitions, Americans of European descent value newness and innovation. They sell or throw away their possessions frequently and replace them with new ones. Generally, people who buy used items (clothes, cars, books, etc.) are viewed as "less fortunate" people who cannot afford to buy these commodities new. The value of newness in possessions can be generalized to other aspects of the lives of Americans of European ancestry: they see change as generally good, leading to development and progress, and they often pursue progress at the expense of stability, continuity, tradition, and heritage (Kohls, 1989).

Technology

As a culture, Americans of European descent are not only technologically oriented but also technologically dependent. Technology has created an extreme of self-sufficiency that makes it possible for a person rarely to ask anything of another in routine daily life (Vargas, 1987). With enough money (or credit), Americans of European descent can buy food transported from all over the world; heat and light their homes; dispose of their waste products; clean their bodies, clothes, and homes; and provide themselves with a variety of high-quality entertainment. Only when a disaster destroys the technologic infrastructure do they realize how dependent their society has become on technology and how this technology acts to distance people from one another. Because technology is so much part of day-today existence, Americans of European descent take for granted technology that would seem magical (not to mention confusing or intimidating) if they were seeing it for the first time.

Directness and Honesty

Americans of European descent generally prefer to communicate directly. In a study of twenty-four families whose children had been diagnosed with a disability, Krahn et al. (1993) asked families to discuss what they liked and disliked about how they were told bad news. Half of families interviewed spontaneously mentioned appreciating information that was "clear, direct, understandable, and detailed." Families did not appreciate having the informer "beat around the bush." When a person uses an indirect approach to giving information, such as using an intermediary to deliver a message, he or she may be considered "manipulative" and "untrustworthy" (Kohls, 1989).

Mobility

Americans of European descent expect to be able to get where whey are going, and be there on time. In fact, their society depends on people being mobile—commuting to work, traveling to business meetings, going across town on an errand, or flying to visit family for the holidays. They also expect everybody else to be equally mobile, sometimes interpreting someone's lack of mobility as lack of motivation.

In this mobile society it is increasingly easy for individuals and families to pick up and move. As a result, family members are often scattered around the country, if not the world. It is rare to find a family in which all the relatives are living in their hometown. Because Americans of European descent value individualism, the ease with which an individual leaves home is viewed positively rather than negatively.

BELIEFS ABOUT HEALTH

Most Americans of European descent believe that illness results from one of three processes: interaction between an external pathogen (e.g., virus, cigarette smoke) and the host (a human body); accidents of development leading to congenital defects; or natural degeneration. These etiologies explain disease as the product of an asocial, amoral process. The patient is seen as the context of the disease, but the patient and the disease are rarely viewed within a larger social context—another manifestation of individualism (Freund and McGuire, 1991). The patient has merely fallen victim to a set of unmediated natural processes that call for technical intervention (Comaroff, 1982).

In keeping with a pragmatic nature, technical intervention has a very no-nonsense approach. They give antibiotics to kill the invading organism, cut out tumors, and stitch up wounds. Treatments are generally concrete and rarely include a metaphysical or spiritual component—the concept of treating an illness with meditation rather than medication is viewed skeptically. As a result of this practical, "what's the bottom line?" approach to life, many, but not all, medical treatments have received rigorous evaluation to determine effectiveness, possible side effects, and cost-benefit ratio before being allowed onto the market. As alternative (generally Eastern, more spiritual) approaches to treatment are being considered by the West, efforts are made to subject them to the same standards.

European-Americans are accustomed to tangible and scientifically proven treatments. They have great respect for American medicine and often assume that it can fix just about anything. The limited availability of treatment and prevention of genetic disease disappoints them.

While many Americans of European descent are skeptical of anything but mainstream Western medicine, medical practices of other cultures or subcultures (e.g., acupuncture and herbal, naturopathic, homeopathic, and holistic approaches) are available and used by Americans of all cultural backgrounds. Health care providers should ascertain if their patients are using such treatments, and whenever possible, incorporate them into the management plan.

As patients, Americans of European descent have certain expectations about how they will be treated during a medical interaction. Because they value autonomy, they expect to participate in their medical care. They will want to be told what will happen to them during an appointment, to have the rationale behind decisions explained to them, and to have opportunities to accept or refuse a test or treatment. If a photograph will be taken as part of the medical record, the practitioner should obtain the patient's or parent's permission. If a physical exam is necessary, teenagers or adults should be allowed to decide whether to have family members present in the room during the examination. Because Americans of European ancestry are time conscious, they appreciate medical appointments that run on time and can accommodate their busy schedules. If delays are unavoidable, patients should be given the option to reschedule the appointment.

Much of modern genetic technology was developed in the United States by Americans of European descent. As a result of their origins, these technologies reflect the values discussed in this chapter. Birth defects and genetic disease, which are viewed as accidents of development, represent a challenge to be overcome with creative, practical, and technical intervention. While it is certainly preferable to cure a birth defect, when this is not possible, many (but not all) Americans of European descent prefer to know during a pregnancy whether their child will have a congenital anomaly. This information may often be obtained through prenatal diagnostic testing, such as amniocentesis, chorionic villus sampling, or ultrasound. The information will allow parents-to-be to make decisions about continuing with or terminating a pregnancy and caring for an affected child after birth. Personal, religious, and moral beliefs, family situation, and perception of the severity of the condition all factor into a family's decision. These factors vary considerably among families, as do the ultimate decisions. Carrier testing and other forms of genetic testing also provide individuals with information they find helpful for making decisions about their future. The fact that many patients of European descent seek out such information about a pregnancy or their own genetic status reflects the value of autonomy and self-determination and the orientation toward the future. They tend to appreciate technology that provides them with such information, although the consequent decisions can be exceedingly difficult and painful—so painful, in fact, that many patients will express ambivalence about the technology they once embraced.

Genetic disease itself represents a challenge to the belief that people create their own future. It is difficult for families to accept that genetic mutation generally does not result from anything that a parent does and that many birth defects appear to be the result of chance. Mothers will often feel guilty that they may have done something wrong and resent that women who had not taken good care of themselves during a pregnancy (e.g., smoked, drank alcohol, used drugs) may nonetheless have normal, healthy babies. Often a family's response to this challenge to their control and autonomy is to do everything medically possible for the child, hoping to cure the problem. Some may even devote time to raising funds for medical research that could eventually find a cure. While this approach often benefits the child and family, it could convey to disabled children they are not accepted by their families. Many families find it helpful to join support groups of other families of children with a similar birth defect or genetic illness: meeting others in the same situation can alleviate feelings of guilt and increase a sense of control over their lives.

While birth defects and disability pose a threat to a sense of autonomy and self-determination, they also threaten the desire for equality. The saying that anyone can grow up to be president seems unlikely in the presence of a child with Down syndrome or other conditions resulting in mental retardation. In recent years, legislation and social movements have increased access to education, buildings, and adaptive equipment for people with all forms of disability. It is hoped that in time and with the aid of technology, a disabled person who has enough initiative and responsibility will be able to accomplish anything. Because technology is better able to minimize the effect of physical defects than those of mental retardation, and because mental ability is required to operate in a technological society, mental retardation is often seen as a worse handicap by Americans of European descent.

Another challenge genetic disease poses to the values of Americans of European descent lies in the familial nature of genetic information. Genetic information, with its implications for extended family, threatens the societal values of autonomy and privacy. Many genetic dilemmas result from the conflict between these values and the fact that the extended family will be affected by, or will potentially benefit from, a person's obtaining personal genetic information. For example, people may learn they carry a genetic disease and know other relatives may be carriers as well. Such people might struggle with the desire to warn their families and yet at the same time not want to disclose their carrier status because the information is personal and because they are concerned others might perceive them as somehow defective. Another dilemma occurs when one person desires testing for a particular gene, but the nature of the test requires that a relative also be tested. This threatens both people's privacy and autonomy, depending on what final decision about testing is reached. Mobility within the culture may obstruct obtaining and disclosing information, as family members may be scattered nationwide and medical care may have been provided at many locations. It is also possible for family members to lose contact completely. An estranged relative may be an important link in obtaining critical information. It is generally accepted that these dilemmas are best handled by discussing the situation and potential outcomes with patients, who can then find their own solution. In this way, patients remain autonomous and maintain a sense of control.

Perhaps the ultimate challenge to the value system of Americans of European descent is death. In facing death, they face losing their autonomy, and there is nothing their affluence, technology, and initiative can do about it. Because death challenges their value system so completely, Americans of European ancestry may avoid this topic whenever possible. As a result, medical discussions regarding death (telling a person of a fatal diagnosis, discussing the reasons to do an autopsy or to store DNA, or planning a death or funeral ritual) may produce socially awkward situations. The health care provider should be sensitive to a family's discomfort without compromising the directness and honesty so clearly appreciated. Autopsies are required by law under some circumstances. When an autopsy is not required by law, a family should have the pros and cons of the autopsy laid out for them. This way the family can make a decision about whether an autopsy will be performed and how extensive the autopsy will be.

Rituals surrounding death and burial reflect the variety of religious and personal beliefs of families of European descent. Families should be consulted throughout the process to ensure that they are comfortable with the decisions that are made. Some families will have very clear ideas about how such rituals should be conducted. Others may be uncertain about how to handle death and funerals, as it is not uncommon for adults to reach their fourth decade without experiencing the death of close family or friends. These families will generally appreciate opportunities to learn about their options in terms of religious services, mementos (especially if a young child has died), and burial or cremation. However, they may feel uncomfortable initiating such discussions.

On the whole, Americans of European descent have great respect for Western medicine and technology. They may be surprised and disappointed when their genetic professional informs them that there is no way to test for, or cure, a certain genetic condition. Despite this common disappointment, genetic professionals can generally develop and maintain a good relationship if they are direct and honest, and if they respect the patient's privacy and autonomy. In such a relationship, most patients of European descent and their families will appreciate and benefit from their contact with a genetic clinic.

CONCLUSION

The culture of Americans of European descent blends the customs and traditions of the initial European immigrants with those of Native Americans and subsequent immigrants from Europe and other continents. This culture continues to change under the influence of continuing immigration, which is now primarily from non-European nations.

While most Americans of European descent share general beliefs about the importance of individualism, equality, and productivity, they will vary in their specific religious beliefs, their views on medical intervention, and their perception of the burden of genetic illness. Because Americans of European ancestry see themselves as unique individuals, they then appreciate it when genetic care providers take the time to understand their personal situation, respect their specific beliefs and values, and communicate with them in a direct yet sensitive manner.

SUMMARY

—Greet people with a handshake.

—Avoid formality, except with older individuals.

—See patients on time when possible, and discuss schedule changes with them.

—Speak directly and honestly, and maintain eye contact throughout the session.

—Before beginning a counseling session, ask the patient to articulate expectations and questions.

—Give the patient opportunities to ask questions during and after a counseling session. Answer these questions thoroughly and respectfully.

—Avoid professional jargon. Explain technical terms in understandable language. Sometimes visual aids are useful.

—Present material at a level appropriate to the patient's ability to comprehend.

—Do not make assumptions about family structure. Confirm all relevant relationships directly with appropriate family members (e.g., do not simply assume that an adult male present with a mother and child is the child's father).

—Encourage patients who have alternative approaches to health care to incorporate as many of their practices as possible into their management.

—If it is necessary to obtain private information, explain why such information is needed before asking personal questions. Assure patients that information obtained during the appointment will be kept confidential, especially private information such as false paternity or previous elective abortions.

—If multiple family members are seen in a clinic, each person should have an opportunity to meet privately with the genetic professional.

—Explain consent forms and give patients the opportunity to review them before signing.

—Make referrals to support groups and provide the family with written materials that are appropriate to their level of understanding.

—Give patients a sense of hope, when appropriate, by discussing current research and reproductive options (e.g., adoption, artificial insemination).

—Allow families to make their own decisions about testing, treatment, and reproductive options. Communicate that you will support whatever decision they make.

—Talk to all adults present. If a patient is from a two-parent household, expect parents to make decisions together.

—Do not make assumptions about religious beliefs, especially those relating to reproduction, abortion, death, and funeral practices. Provide families with appropriate information and discuss all possible options with them.

REFERENCES

Caudill, W. 1976. The cultural and interpersonal context of everyday health and illness in Japan and America. In Leslie, C. M. (ed.), *Asian Medical Systems: A Comparative Study,* pp. 159 77. Berkeley: University of California Press.

Comaroff, J. 1982. Medicine: Symbol and ideology. In Wright, P., and Treacher, A. (eds.), *The Problem of Medical Knowledge,* pp. 49–67. Edinburgh: Edinburgh University Press.

Davis-Floyd, R. 1994. *Birth as an American Rite of Passage.* Berkeley: University of California Press.

de Tocqueville, A. C. 1969. *Democracy in America.* New York: Doubleday.

Freund, P. E. S., and McGuire, M. B. 1991. The social construction of medical knowledge. In Freund, P. E. S., and McGuire, M. B. (eds.), *Health, Illness, and the Social Body: A Critical Sociology,* pp. 203–29. New York: Prentice Hall.

Hanson, M. J. 1992. Families with Anglo-European roots. In Lynch, E. W., and Hanson, M. J. (eds.), *Developing Cross-Cultural Competence: A Guide for Working with Young Children and Their Families,* pp. 65–86. Baltimore: Paul H. Brookes.

Kohls, L. R. 1989. Why do Americans act like that? *On Beyond War* (October). Newsletter. Palo Alto, Calif.

Krahn, G. L., Hallum, A., and Kime, C. 1993. Are there good ways to give "bad news"? *Pediatrics* 91:578–82.

Lakoff, G., and Johnson, M. 1980. *Metaphors We Live By.* Chicago: University of Chicago Press.

Mead, F. S. 1990. *Handbook of Denominations in the United States,* 9th ed. Nashville: Abingdon.

Rothman, B. K. 1989. *Recreating Motherhood: Ideology and Technology in Patriarchal Society.* New York: W. W. Norton.

Vargas, M. O. 1987. Tradition of nontradition: Our cultural blind spot. *Birth Defects* 23:122–32.

Wong, J., and Banerian, J. 1980. American-Vietnamese cross-cultural information. *Indochinese Community Health and Education Project Cultural Awareness Training Manual,* pp. 26–32. San Diego: Indochinese Community Health and Education Project.

2

Latino Culture

Elena Lopez-Rangel, M.D., M.Sc.

The term *Hispanic* originates from the Latin word *hispanicus,* or *Hispanica* (Iberian peninsula), and refers to the people, speech, or culture of Spain, Portugal, and Latin America. Since 1970 the U.S. Bureau of the Census has used *Hispanic* as a generic term to identify individuals of Spanish origin or descent. For census purposes, a Hispanic person is defined as a native, or resident, of the southwestern United States, descended from Spaniards who settled before annexation (U.S. Bureau of the Census, 1970). Persons of Hispanic descent may have recently moved to the United States, or their families may have lived here for centuries. Even though the cultural and historic roots of Hispanic people are, in fact, found in the Iberian peninsula, some authors (Perez-Stable, 1987; Gimenez, 1989) have objected to the Hispanic label on the basis that this term implies a heritage restricted to Spain.

Latino is the Latin word for "Spanish," and the root of the prefix for the American continent south of the United States, Latin America. Some authors (Perez-Stable, 1987; Gimenez, 1989) have considered that the term *Latino* better reflects the union of Spanish, indigenous, and African cultures that are part of Latin America. This term is used as a generic ethnic label by the American Public Health Association.

This chapter uses the term *Latino* except in cases in which the U.S. Bureau of the Census or the U.S. Department of Health, Education, and Welfare is cited. Using the term *Hispanic* allows for a better review of the demographic statistics of Latinos in the United States. As the term *Latino* more truly reflects the melding of the cultures that emerged in Latin America, it has been selected for use in this chapter.

The Latino population is not homogeneous. It is made up of several distinct populations that differ in national origin, culture, race, and ethnicity. The literature divides the U.S. Hispanic / Latino population into five subgroups: Mexican American, Puerto Rican, Cuban American, Central or South American, and "other" Hispanics / Latinos. This classification is oversimplified, because there is considerable overlap among the different groups and because there is substantial ethnic and cultural diversity within each of the regions used to define the groups.

HISTORY

Native Americans, Spaniards, and African natives have all contributed to contemporary Latino populations (Hanis et al., 1991). American Indians are thought to have arrived on the North American continent via the Bering Strait from Asia. Christopher Columbus arrived in the West Indies in 1492. After that, a continuous flow of Spanish explorers settled in the Americas. By 1915, the Spaniards had occupied an extensive territory, including the Canary Islands, most of the Caribbean Islands, most of Central and South America, and all of Mexico, including the territory that is now Texas, California, Utah, Nevada, parts of New Mexico, Arizona, Colorado, and Wyoming (Samora and Vandel-Simon, 1977).

In Mexico, contact with the Spaniards began in 1519, with the arrival of the Spanish explorer Hernan Cortés. The initial contact was with the coastal Indians of Veracruz. The Spaniards continued westward to the center of Mexico, finally settling in what is now Mexico City. In Mexico, the mixture began as Mexicans and Aztec Indian chiefs offered their daughters as gifts to the newcomers. Very early during the conquest, a *castas,* or caste system, arose. The population was divided into sixteen racial categories by parenthood, skin color, and the "amount" of Spanish blood a person had (Samora and Vandel-Simon, 1977).

With the Spanish conquerors came a new language, religion, and government, as well as the slave industry. The importation of slaves from Africa resulted in a small but significant black mixture. The contribution made by natives to the population in all of Latin America was limited by the devastation of imported diseases and war (Samora and Vandel-Simon, 1977). In 1821 Mexico became independent from Spain.

Until 1848, Mexico controlled much of the Southwestern United States. In 1848 Mexico agreed, in the Treaty of Guadalupe, to withdraw from this area. This treaty brought an end to the U.S.-Mexican War.

In Puerto Rico, as in Mexico, slaves from West Africa were "imported." Their contribution is much more noticeable in Puerto Rico, where integration and intermarriage were freely accepted (Fitzpatrick, 1971).

In Cuba, the conquest began in 1510, and the native population was decimated early. Later, and mainly because of the sugar cane plantations, many African slaves were imported and a fair amount of African, native, and Spanish intermixture occurred (Alum and Mantrisa, 1977).

DEMOGRAPHICS

According to the U.S. Bureau of the Census, an estimated 22 million Hispanics now live in the United States. The majority, 63 percent, are Mexican American, 12 percent are Puerto Rican, 5 percent are Cuban American, 10 percent are Central and South American, and 8 percent are referred to as "other Hispanics." Most Hispanics (87 percent) live in urban areas, and 82.9 percent are concentrated in eight states, with California and Texas containing 51.6 percent of the total Hispanic population in the United States (tables 2.1 and 2.2).

Recent statistics show that Hispanics have a lower income, a shorter life expectancy, more crowded housing conditions, fewer professional jobs, and a lower proportion of high school graduates than the U.S. population as a whole (U.S. Bureau of the Census, 1989). In 1985, the median annual income was $19,000 for a Hispanic family, compared to $26,000 for the general population. Cuban Americans have the highest level of both education and income among Hispanics (Mendoza et al., 1991; Frank-Stromberg, 1991). Twenty-five percent of Mexican Americans and 38 percent of Puerto Ricans live below the poverty line, compared to 10 percent of the non-Hispanic white population. Thirty-three percent of the Hispanic population, most of whom work, have no health insurance. This is a substantial figure, particularly as compared to the 15 percent of uninsured non-Hispanics residing in the United States (Council on Scientific Affairs, 1991; U.S. Bureau

Table 2.1. Largest Increase in Latino Population

State	1990 Population	Increase from 1980 (%)	Percentage of Population
Rhode Island	45,752	132.2	4.6
Nevada	124,419	130.9	10.4
Massachusetts	287,549	102.8	1.0
Virginia	160,288	100.7	2.6

Source: Data from 1990 Census

Table 2.2. Highest Concentration of Latino Population

State	1990 Population	Increase from 1980 (%)	Percentage of Population
New Mexico	579,224	21.4	38.2
California	7,667,938	69.2	25.8
Texas	4,339,905	45.4	25.5
Arizona	588,338	56.2	18.8
Colorado	424,302	24.9	12.9

Source: Data from 1990 Census

of the Census, 1989; Solis et al., 1990). The average Hispanic is less well educated than the average non-Hispanic American: 13.5 percent of Hispanics have less than five years of schooling, compared with 2 percent of the overall population.

The Hispanic population is the fastest-growing minority group in the United States (see table 2.1). The number of Hispanic persons residing in the United States has been growing five times as fast as any other ethnic group (Mendoza et al., 1991). Since 1980, the non-Hispanic population has increased only 8 percent (Rich, 1989), while the Hispanic population has increased 39 percent, due to immigration and high birth rates. The fertility rate among Hispanics (97 of 1,000) is higher than that of the general population (65 of 1,000). Moreover, Hispanic women give birth at younger ages and tend to have more children (an average of three). The median age of the Hispanic population is twenty-five, with 48 percent of all Hispanics under the age of thirty-five. This means that a large number of women are currently of reproductive age and the high birth rate can be expected to continue. An estimated 22 million Hispanic persons now live in the United States. By the year 2000 there will be about 25 million Hispanics; they will be the single largest minority group in the United States (Balcazar and Oayama, 1991).

Every country in Latin America has different dates for specific national holidays. Many of the holidays are religious days of observance, since the majority of Latinos are Roman Catholic. African and indigenous people's religious / supernatural beliefs have also strongly influenced the practice of religion among Latinos. However, because Latinos are in diverse geographic areas, religious beliefs and practices are not homogeneous.

In Mexico, Independence Day is celebrated on September 16, but December 12, "Day of the Virgin of Guadalupe," is just as important. On this day, Mexican Americans may visit church and bring flower arrangements to place before the statue of the Virgin Mary. Individuals may also pray to the Virgin Mary to cure their child of a disability.

An important holiday to remember is Lent, or *Cuaresma*. This is a period of penitence and fasting observed in the forty weekdays from Ash Wednesday *(Miercoles de Ceniza)* to Easter *(Pascua)*, and it changes every year with the Easter calendar. On Ash Wednesday, families attend mass and receive an ash mark on their foreheads. Although no longer required by the Catholic Church, many Latino families follow an old tradition that forbids them from eating meat on Fridays and during Cuaresma.

Maundy Thursday *(Jueves Santo)*, Good Friday (*Viernes Santo*), Saturday *(Sabado de Gloria)*, and Sunday *(Domingo de Resurreccion)* are important to keep in mind. These are times for remembering the death of Jesus Christ. Families usually do not socialize on these days. November 2 is Day of the Dead, reserved for commemorating the lives of deceased family members. The family may visit the cemetery where relatives are buried and bring food and flowers to place on their graves. This day is considered not a sad occasion but a joyous time. Christmas is celebrated on December 24 and is a very significant holiday. (Also see chapter 10, on Christians.)

Not all Latinos are Catholic. Other religious beliefs and denominations such as Protestant, Baptist, and Jewish, have followers in Latino countries. The Roman Catholic Church has restrictions regarding artificial means of birth control. It forbids abortion and permits only natural methods of birth control, such as "coitus interruptus" (Noonan, 1986), the rhythm method, or abstinence. Consequently, prenatal diagnostic procedures (amniocentesis, chorionic villus sampling) are often refused because of their association with abortion. However, some individuals may disagree with church policies, so health care providers should not make any assumptions about an individual's choice regarding prenatal diagnosis. Diversity rather than uniformity influences choices and decisions.

FAMILY

Hispanic families are, on average, larger than non-Hispanic families. Fifty-four percent of Hispanic households consist of four or more people, while in the general population, only 28 percent of families are that large.

The Latino family structure is patriarchal. The father makes the decisions, while the mother handles the running of the home (Lawson, 1990; Burr and Mutchler, 1992). Immediate and extended family members participate in every decision. This characteristic has been called *familismo* (Perez-Stable, 1987; Kirkman-Liff and Mondragon, 1991). *Familismo* emphasizes interdependence over independence, affiliation over individualism, and cooperation over confrontation. This means that Latinos have extended loyalties to all members of their family. This loyalty will sometimes extend beyond the family, as well.

Padrinos (godparents), for example, often participate in a decision that involves their *ahijado* (godchild). The *padrinos* are usually chosen before the child is born and may be family members or close friends of the parents. In Catholic families, they take the child to be baptized and make a vow to raise him or her in the Catholic faith. They are also expected to look after the child if the parents should become ill or die. It is very clear from the family structure that if a Latino is faced with an important medical decision to make alone, he or she is placed in a difficult situation. Counselors should allow the patient to consult with the family. This will reduce the anxiety caused by the decision and will help establish a trusting relationship (Lawson, 1990).

Latinos consider children an essential part of the family. The loss of a child, or even of a pregnancy, represents a loss of expectations and hope for the future. When counseling for death, miscarriage, or the termination of a pregnancy, a practitioner must consider the influence of the culture on the expression of grief and ability to handle particular situations. Latino concepts of death and the afterlife are deeply rooted in Roman Catholicism (Lawson, 1990) and need to be addressed appropriately.

Latino families are very tightly knit and revolve around the development and activities of the children. The studies by Mary (1990) reveal reactions to having a child with a handicap by African American, Caucasian, and Latino mothers. Latino mothers displayed a sense of sacrifice, whereas African American and Caucasian mothers did not. This reaction was found to be even more significant when the family was of lower socioeconomic status. Additionally, in twenty Latino families studied, seven of the fathers were in total denial about their child's disability. While spouses may accept the disability, they deny the prognosis and may have unrealistic expectations for the future care the child will need. Spousal denial was reported in only two of the twenty Caucasian and African American mothers studied.

Latino families have a unique view of adoption. If the parents of a child were to die, it would be appropriate and expected for the grandmother, aunt, older sister, or godmother to take over the role of the deceased parents. However, this situation is viewed not as adoption, per se, but rather as one of the roles of the extended family. Adoptions outside of the family are rare.

COMMUNICATION

Language is critical to the understanding of culture. Many Latinos speak Spanish, but accents and "regionalisms" vary from country to country (Thorngren, 1990). In the United States, some individuals speak Spanish with an English accent because acculturation was so important that Spanish was forbidden in the household. Spanish is spoken in 5 percent of all homes in the United States, but if an American Latino speaks English, do not assume that he or she can also read and write in English—or in Spanish, for that matter.

Studies have shown that Latinos prefer Spanish as the language for an interview (Kirkman-Liff and Mondragon, 1991). A study of more than two thousand Latinos, ages eighteen and older, in twenty-one different metropolitan areas across the United States, found that more than half of the respondents felt more comfortable speaking in Spanish than in English (Korzenny and Schiff, 1987).

Latino families who speak English may not be familiar with medical terms. If a Spanish-speaking counselor or physician is not available, the use of an interpreter is advised. Interpreters are often necessary, not only to exchange information, but also to help both the counselor and patient understand the finer shades of meaning. Professional interpreters may be well accepted, but using a stranger from the waiting room, or a child, may be seen as a loss of the privacy and dignity of the family. Under these circumstances, the patient will be unlikely to reveal private information. Borrego, Chavez, and Titley (1982) and Atkinson et al. (1989) also found that patients expressed greater preference for interpreters of the same sex and ethnic group.

BELIEFS ABOUT HEALTH

The term *curanderismo,* or folk healing, comes from the Spanish word *curar,* which means "to heal." Curanderismo is the treatment of a variety of ailments with a combination of psychosocial interventions, herbs, potions, and religion (Chesney et al., 1980; Kraewski-Jaime, 1991). The practice of curanderismo is a mix of Judeo-Christian religious beliefs, early Arabic medicine and health practices, Native American herbal knowledge, and, more recently, modern psychology and scientific medicine (Trotter and Chavira, 1981; Kraewski-Jaime, 1991).

The three most common beliefs for what causes illness in curanderismo are: (1) natural and supernatural forces, (2) imbalances of heat and cold, and (3) emotions. Cleft lip and palate, for example, are commonly believed to be caused by maternal exposure to supernatural forces during a lunar eclipse. To prevent clefting, pregnant women exposed to an eclipse will wear a belt, from which keys hang directly over the womb, for the remainder of the pregnancy. This will keep the child "locked in" and supposedly safe from harmful supernatural forces (Abril, 1977; Maduro, 1983).

The "evil eye" (curse) is another example of supernatural forces being considered the cause of illness. Someone who admires a child or gives a covetous look, without touching him or her, may be said to cast an "evil eye" *(mal de ojo).* It is believed that to relieve a child of the ill effects of an evil eye, the person who cast the "spell" must touch the child. Some believe that another way to relieve the ailing child is to attach a nutshell to a bracelet, which is then worn by the child. The shell purportedly draws the evil inside itself, protecting the child (Chavira, 1975; Abril, 1977; Maduro, 1983).

Some believe that people can bring on disease through witchcraft, or *brujeria.* This is commonly believed to cause all types of congenital anomalies (Roeder, 1988). *Mal aire,* "cold" or "bad air," is said to cause pain, cramping, facial twitching, and paralysis in children and adults by creating an imbalance of hot and cold. Many mothers are hesitant to take their children from a warm room into the cold, especially infants who have just awakened. It is important to keep an infant covered during an examination to prevent mal aire (Clark, 1970; Roeder, 1988).

It is believed that strong emotions can cause symptoms, which include fatigue, insomnia, and hallucinations. These illnesses are commonly known as *susto,* or fright, and are well recognized by folk healers. Treatments include sweeping the patient's body with branches and herbs while the patient lies on the floor, arms outstretched in the sign of a cross (Abril, 1977; Maduro, 1983; Roeder, 1988). It is thought, for example, that in an earthquake, pregnant women might be frightened into premature labor or may even miscarry. A very strong earthquake might cause the baby to turn to a breech position.

Many Latino people perceive illness as a state of physical discomfort. If a patient has a strong body, with the ability to maintain a normal activity level and no persistent pain or discomfort, he or she is presumed to be healthy (Abril, 1977). This concept of health may make the prevention of disease through genetic counseling difficult to convey and understand.

A *curandero* is a person who practices curanderismo. He or she has the "gift" of healing, and usually lives in the community and shares the experiences, language, and socioeconomic status of his or her patients. The curandero is believed to be gifted, and holds knowledge that has been handed down from generation to generation. Curanderos are always available for the community they live in. They provide valuable counseling, using their knowledge of the patient's family and background to give advice that fits the particular social, economic, and cultural needs. *Curanderos* use the family as a natural support system.

Another type of folk healer is a *sobador,* who treats illness with massages or rubbing. He or she will rub the patient's body with herbal oils. Sobadores are used almost exclusively in muscular or skeletal disorders. However, in some cases infertile women may consult a sobador because of the belief that infertility is associated with a "fallen or twisted uterus." In these cases, the abdomen is massaged with oil until "the uterus is put back into place" (Abril, 1977; Maduro, 1983).

Many Latino families may consult a folk healer before considering a visit to a medical doctor. It is important not to generalize and say that all Latino families consult with curanderos. Factors such as cultural orientation, degree of acculturation, ability to pay, and whether an individual has had good or bad prior experiences with medical practitioners will all play a role in whether a person visits a curandero (Higginbotham, Trevino, and Ray, 1990). In most cases, the folk healer has known the family for years, speaks their language, and does not give orders for care, but makes suggestions, leaving the family in a position to choose the treatment, and thereby retain a sense of control (Abril, 1977; Maduro, 1983). Latino families find the curanderos to be more compassionate and accepting of traditional beliefs and practices than medical doctors (Clark, 1970). It is common, however, for Latino families to use both folk and conventional medicine to treat disease (Thorrey, 1986).

The literature on folk medicine suggests that the choice of conventional care and / or folk medicine depends on the symptom. Chesney et al. (1982) found that more than half of the forty families in their study would go to a curandero in cases of nausea, vomiting, stomach pain, or diarrhea. The same families sought traditional medical advice for symptoms such as earaches, shortness of breath, pain in the chest, blood in the stool, seizures, and eye problems. Latino families were more likely to seek traditional medical help for anxiety, while they almost always consulted a curandero for depression.

Beliefs in folk healing cannot be generalized to all Latino groups, or even to all members of one Latino group. In a study of Mexican American folk medicine, Chesney et al. (1980) found that between 20 and 30 percent of their sample did not believe in folk medicine and that Latinos of lower socioeconomic status tended to rely more heavily on folk healers. However, these folk beliefs and practices may vary from generation to generation and depend mostly on the level of adaptation to the Anglo-American culture.

In addition to relying on folk healers, many Latinos look to home remedies to treat illnesses. Home remedies are inexpensive natural herb products that are used for everything from tuberculosis to migraine headaches. The common belief is that one requires a balance between hot and cold to remain healthy. Therefore, hot diseases are treated with cold elements, while cold diseases are treated with heat. This restores the body's temperature balance. For example, burns must be treated with ice, colds with hot foods (Abril, 1977; Maduro, 1983; Ripley, 1986).

IMPLICATIONS FOR GENETIC SERVICES

Whenever possible, health care practitioners should ascertain a family's country of origin before the counseling session. Each country has its distinct national culture and patients will appreciate being properly referred to as being Mexican, Colombian, Salvadorean.

Latino patients view physicians as important authority figures (Perez-Stable, 1987). Although expecting an authoritative expert, Latinos also expect a friend with whom they can talk openly. *Personalismo,* or formal friendliness, is the description for one who can provide professional services, speaking with authority and, at the same time, offering warmth and friendliness. This establishes a relationship between people, not with the institution (Padilla, Ruiz, and Alvarez, 1976; Chavez, 1979). Most Latino patients do not readily accept the impersonality that often accompanies modern Western medicine (Perez-Stable, 1987).

In Latino cultures, *respeto* (respect) is expected. This term encompasses the expectation that the patient will demonstrate deference to the physician. The physician, in turn, is expected to show appreciation for the patient, whose concern deserves serious consideration (Erzinger, 1991). Respeto begins with the very first contact between a patient and a physician. Latinos are less physically distant in personal interactions and are accustomed to frequent physical contact. Handshakes and embraces between friends are the norm (Ingram, 1991). Practitioners should greet the most senior male first, followed by the most senior female. Not offering this greeting is considered rude (Quesada, 1976; Perez-Stable, 1987). A pat on the hand or a clasp on the arm is taken as a sign of concern and good will (Hardwood, 1981). Traditionally, Latinos have been taught to avoid eye contact with authority figures (such as a physician) as a sign of respect. This behavior should not be interpreted as disinterest in communication (Ingram, 1991). Latinos may sit closer than other patients during the session. Sitting too far from the patient may be perceived as detachment.

Being *simpatico* is another characteristic that Latinos expect from physicians and counselors. This word has no equivalent in English. It refers to a personal quality of an individual who is likable, attractive, fun to be with, and easygoing. An individual who is simpatico has an ability to share others' feelings, behaves with dignity and respect toward others, and strives for harmony in interpersonal relations (Triandis et al., 1984). The friendly role of the curandero within Latino communities has led Latino patients to have similar expectations of the more traditional medical practitioner. Latino families assume that the physician will take time to engage in conversation and be friendly and supportive, and they may interpret the absence of special interest as a lack of overall concern, or even as prejudice against them (Hardwood, 1981).

As with many other ethnic groups, Latinos exhibit modesty. Measures to preserve privacy should be observed at all times, with care taken to expose as little of the body as possible during examinations and treatments. This is especially important for pregnant women. If the physician doing the examination is male, it may be necessary for the husband to be in the room.

Prenatal diagnostic procedures (amniocentesis, chorionic villus sampling) may not be highly utilized. Most Catholic Latino families will not consider abortion as an option, and may perceive the suggestion as an insult. Since termination of an abnormal pregnancy may not be an option, the concept of prenatal diagnosis may be viewed as unnecessary. The counselor or physician should take special care when broaching this subject. Catholicism holds that illness or death is "God's will." Another common belief is that many illnesses develop because of God's disapproval of the patient's behavior. According to Abril (1977), this belief is more prevalent in cases of congenital anomalies of undetermined etiology. Although it is important, at such times, to inform patients that they did nothing wrong and to explain that a certain number of infants are born with birth defects, the concept may not be fully accepted.

The definition of disabilities may vary among Latino groups. Mental retardation may not be seen as a handicap to some if the individual, for example, can work in the fields alongside other family members. However, a limb deficiency would be a major disability in this same situation. Among other families, where academic or intellectual pursuits are the norm, mental retardation may be an important issue.

Genetic and biological concepts are sometimes difficult to understand during the stress of counseling. Visual aids and follow-up letters may be useful. When giving out printed handouts, ascertain if literature in Spanish or English is more appropriate.

Marriage between first cousins does not often occur since it is discouraged by social and religious mores. Nonpaternity may occur and should be dealt with on an individual basis. In classic Hispanic culture, nonpaternity was rare; however, teens and younger women living in the United States have more sexual freedom than in the past.

Although the family is the mainstay of support, the Latino community in the United States has a large network of community organizations for support. Know what groups are available in each community. These groups may be helpful to the family, since psychological counseling may not be readily accepted.

In situations concerning the health care of infants and children, it is important to remember that, even though the decision is made by the family members as a group, the mother will probably be the one to provide most, if not all, of the care for a handicapped child. If the mother works or is unable to take care of the child, this responsibility will fall on one of the grandmothers, the godmother, or even the eldest sister. She will be responsible for feeding, dressing, teaching, and locating appropriate community resources for rehabilitation or ongoing treatment and therapy for the child (Maduro, 1983). Consequently, it is essential to address the female caregiver when discussing the care of a child.

Latinos tend to express emotions openly when faced with a crisis or illness. Remaining calm when confronted with traumatic news is considered culturally inappropriate behavior (Perez-Stable, 1987; Erzinger, 1991). However, open discussion of feelings is discouraged, particularly if the openness is with individuals outside the family.

It is important to be familiar with customs surrounding death and funerals, family life patterns, lines of authority, roles of family members during periods of grief, the amount of help available, and the family's expectations of health care professionals during death and periods of grief. For example, baptizing a baby who is not expected to live for very long is very important. In urgent situations, it is not even necessary to wait for a priest; any Catholic or Christian person can baptize a child by anointing the forehead with water, making the sign of the cross and saying, "In the name of the Father, and the Son, and the Holy Ghost, I baptize you." This will ensure that the baby's soul will be blessed and go to heaven (Abril, 1977). This may be requested by some families and must be done as soon as the baby is born if he or she is not expected to live. Most Catholic Latino families will not allow autopsy and will want to hold a mass, burial, and/or cremation for the dead. (See chapter 10, on Christians.) However, the importance or necessity of an autopsy should be clearly and objectively explained to the family.

Mandas, pledges to God or a patron saint, are made to ensure the welfare of an individual in any dangerous circumstance. This is an especially common practice among pregnant women. The woman may promise, for example, not to cut her infant's hair until a specific age and only after making a visit to a special chapel or church (Abril, 1977).

Immediate and extended family and close friends are primary sources of help in cases of disease, death, and even the birth of a child with a disability. Disclosing an illness to strangers, however, is often a shameful or painful experience. This particular situation becomes very important when dealing with inherited disorders. Latinos may be hesitant to talk to other family members for fear of losing their *dignidad* (dignity) (Perez-Stable, 1987).

Latinos have a higher than average incidence of diabetes, neural tube defects, and cancers of the gall bladder, liver, pancreas, cervix, and stomach (Padilla, 1984; Hanis et al., 1991). Cervical and stomach cancers occur twice as frequently among Latinos as among non-Latino whites. Prostate cancer is the most common type of cancer seen in Latino males, while breast and colorectal cancers are the most common in Latino females (Frank-Stromberg, 1991).

CONCLUSION

It is critical to remember that the value placed on manners and courtesy extends to personal relationships. Health care professionals should ensure that relations appear harmonious even when they aren't. A couple will never openly discuss differences of opinion, especially in front of a counselor or physician. Therefore, when difficult decisions need to be made, a couple should be allowed time for private discussion (Triandis et al., 1984).

In view of the importance given to personalismo, respeto, and being simpatico, it is best for Latino patients to deal with the same physician most of the time. Among Latinos, rotating staff is not an effective way to encourage patient participation in health care (Thorngren, 1990). Therefore, a family should be contacted and recontacted by the same genetic counselor. Likewise, the counselor can inform the family / couple that they may phone with specific questions or concerns.

SUMMARY

—Greet the eldest male first. Shake hands and establish rapport with family by asking about family, etc.

—Even if the family / couple speaks English, inquire if an interpreter is needed for medical terminology. Avoid using strangers and children as interpreters; the same sex and ethnic group would be most effective.

—Speak directly to the mother or other females about care of the children, since this is their responsibility.

—Although many Latinos are Catholic, prenatal diagnostic testing should be offered.

—Disclosure of carrier status or a child's disability to other family members may be difficult because the family views it as a loss of dignity.

—Disability may be defined by the function in the family and community, not by medical definitions.

—Family members participate in all decisions, so allow couples and patients time to consult with other family members.

—The loss of a pregnancy is viewed like the loss of a child.

—Referral to community resources is important.

—Adoption should be mentioned when appropriate, although adoption rarely occurs outside the family.

—The concept of prevention of disease may be difficult to understand because if a person is healthy and has no discomfort, he or she is presumed to be healthy and there is no need for intervention.

—Families / couples may use both folk healers and Western physicians. It may be helpful to ask what other treatments have been sought and what they believe to be the cause of their particular problem.

—Ask what country the patient is from and refer to individuals as Mexican, Guatemalan, etc.

—Visual aids may be helpful in explaining genetic concepts.

—Ascertain whether the family / patient wishes to receive printed handouts in English or in Spanish.

—If the patient / family needs to be seen more than once, it is important to have the same counselor or health provider. If a new counselor or provider will be working , introduce him or her to the family.

—Latinos tend to express emotions openly when faced with a crisis. Allow time for such display. A calm touch of support would be welcome.

—Many Latinos will avoid confrontation and disagreement by not expressing doubts or asking questions. Inform patients that questions are expected.

—Do not express negative feelings directly; use an indirect approach.

REFERENCES

Abril, I. F. 1977. Mexican American folk beliefs: How they affect health care. *American Journal of Maternal and Child Nursing* 2:168–73.

Alum, R. A., and Mantrisa, F. P. 1977. Cuban and American values: A synoptic comparison. *Mosaic: Hispanic Subcultural Values: Similarities and Differences,* pp. 184–202. Institute for Intercultural Relations and Ethnic Studies. New Brunswick, N.J.: Rutgers University.

Atkinson, D. R., Poston, W. C., Furlong, M. J., and Mercado, P. 1989. Ethnic group preferences for counselor characteristics. *Journal of Counseling Psychology* 36:68–72.

Balcazar, H., and Oayama, C. 1991. Interpretive views on Hispanics' perinatal problems of low birthweight and prenatal care. *Public Health Reports* 106:420–26.

Borrego, R. L., Chavez, E. L., and Titley, R. W. 1982. Effect of counselor technique on Mexican American and Anglo-American self-disclosure and counselor perception. *Journal of Counseling Psychology* 29:538–41.

Burr, J. A., and Mutchler, J. E. 1992. The living arrangements of unmarried elderly Hispanic females. *Demography* 29:93–112.

Chavez, N. 1979. Mexican American expectations of treatment, role of self and therapists: Effects on utilization of mental health services. In Martin, P. P. (ed.), *La Frontera Perspective: Providing Health Services to Mexican-Americans*. Tucson, Ariz.: Old Pueblo Printers.

Chavira, P. 1975. *Curanderismo: An Optimal Health Care System*. Edinburg, Tex.: Pan American University.

Chesney, A. P., Thompson, B. L., Guevara, A., Vela, A., and Schottsteadt, M. F. 1980. Mexican American folk medicine: Implications for the family physician. *Journal of Family Practice* 11:567–74.

Chesney, A. P., Chavira, J. A., Hall, R. P., and Gary, H. E., Jr. 1982. Barriers to medical care of Mexican Americans: The role of social class, acculturation, and social isolation. *Medical Care* 20:883–91.

Clark, M. 1970. *Health in the Mexican American Culture: A Community Study*. 2d ed. Berkeley: University of California Press.

Council on Scientific Affairs. 1991. Hispanic health in the United States. *Journal of the American Medical Association* 265:248–52.

Erzinger S. 1991. Communication between Spanish-speaking patients and their doctors in medical encounters. *Culture, Medicine, and Psychiatry* 15:91–110.

Fitzpatrick, J. P. 1971. Puerto Ricans: The meaning of migration to the mainland. In Gordon, M. M. (ed.), *Ethnic Groups in American Life Series*, pp. 251–57. Englewood Cliffs, N.J.: Prentice Hall.

Frank-Stromberg, M. 1991. Changing demographics in the United States: Implications for health professionals. *Cancer* 67:1772–78.

Gimenez, M. E. 1989. Latino / "Hispanic": Who needs a name? The case against standardized terminology. *International Journal of Health Services* 19:557–71.

Hanis, C. L., Hewett-Emmett, D., Bertin, T. K., and Schull, W. J. 1991. Origins of U.S. Hispanics: Implications for diabetes. *Diabetes Care* 14:618–27.

Hardwood, A. 1981. *Ethnicity and Medical Care*. Cambridge: Harvard University Press.

Higginbotham, J. C., Trevino, F. M., and Ray, L. A. 1990. Utilization of curanderos by Mexican Americans, Prevalence and Predictors: Findings from HHANES, 1982–84. *American Journal of Public Health* 80:32–35.

Ingram, C. A. 1991. How can we become more aware of culturally specific body language and use this awareness therapeutically? *Journal of Psychosocial Nursing and Mental Health Services* 29:38–41.

Kirkman-Liff, B., and Mondragon, D. 1991. Language and interview: Relevance for research of southwest Hispanics. *American Journal of Public Health* 81:1399–1404.

Korzenny, F., and Schiff, E. 1987. Hispanic perceptions of communication discrimination. *Hispanic Journal of Behavioral Science* 9:33–48.

Kraewski-Jaime, E. R. 1991. Folk healing among Mexican American families as a consideration in the delivery of child welfare and child health services. *Child Welfare* 70:157–67.

Lawson, L. V. 1990. Culturally sensitive support for grieving parents. *American Journal of Maternal and Child Nursing* 15:76–79.

Maduro, R. 1983. Curanderismo and Latino views of disease and curing. *Western Journal of Medicine* 139:868–74.

Mary, N. 1990. Reactions of black, Hispanic and white mothers to having a child with handicaps. *Mental Retardation* 28:1–5.

Mendoza, F. S., Ventura, S. J., Valdez, R. B., Castillo, R. O., Saldivar, L. E., Baisden, K., and Martorell, R. 1991. Selected measures of health status for Mexican-American, mainland Puerto Rican, and Cuban-American children. *Journal of the American Medical Association* 265:227–32.

Noonan, J. T., Jr. 1986. *Contraception: A History of the Treatment by the Catholic Theologians and Canonists.* Cambridge: Harvard University Press.

Padilla, A., Ruis, R., and Alvarez, R. 1976. Delivery of community mental health services to Spanish speaking / surnamed populations. 1976. In Alvarez, R. (ed.), *Delivery of Services for Latino Community Mental Health.* Monograph no. 2. University of California, Los Angeles. Los Angeles: Spanish-Speaking Mental Health Development Program.

Padilla, F. M. 1984. On the nature of Latin ethnicity. *Social Science Quarterly* 84:65–71.

Perez-Stable, E. 1987. Issues in Latino health care. *Western Journal of Medicine* 146:213–18.

Quesada, G. M. 1976. Language and communication barriers for health care delivery to a minority group. *Social Science and Medicine* 10:323–27.

Rich, S. 1989. Hispanic population of the U.S. growing fastest: Census Bureau puts total at 20.1 million. *Washington Post,* 12 Oct.

Ripley, G. D. 1986. Mexican American folk remedies: Their place in health care. *Texas Medicine* 82:41–44.

Roeder, B. 1988. Chicano folk medicine from Los Angeles, California. In *Folklore and Mythology.* Los Angeles: University of California Publications.

Samora, J., and Vandel-Simon, P. 1977. *A History of the Mexican American People.* South Bend, Ind.: University of Notre Dame Press.

Solis, J. M., Marks, G., Garcia, M., and Shelton, D. 1990. Acculturation, access to care, and use of preventive services by Hispanics: Findings from HHANES, 1982–84. *American Journal of Public Health* 80:11–19.

Thorngren, M. 1990. *Health Care of Hispanic Populations,* pp. 39–45. Birth Defects Original Article Series, no. 26. Washington, D.C.: March of Dimes.

Thorrey, P. 1986. *Witch Doctors and Psychiatry.* Northvale, N.J.: Jason Aaronson, pp. 155–68.

Triandis, H. C., Marin, G., Lisansky, J., and Betancourt, H. 1984. Simpatica as a cultural script of Hispanics. *Journal of Personality and Social Psychology* 47:1363–75.

Trotter, R., and Chavira, J. A. 1981. *Curanderismo.* Athens: University of Georgia Press.

U.S. Bureau of the Census. 1970. *The Hispanic Population in the U.S.* Current Population Reports. Washington, D.C.: GPO.

———. 1989. Money, Income, and Poverty Status in the United States. Current Population Report, ser. P-60, no. 166. Washington, D.C.: GPO.

———. 1991. 1990 Census Results. *Statistical Bulletin* 72:21–27.

Wilson, M. G., Chan, L. S., and Herbert, W. S. 1992. Birth prevalence of Down syndrome in a predominantly Latino population: A fifteen-year study. *Teratology* 45:285–92.

3

African American Culture

Joseph Telfair, Dr.P.H., M.S.W., M.P.H., and
Kermit B. Nash, Ph.D.

Americans of African descent are often perceived as a homogeneous group, but in fact are diversified according to their degree of assimilation into the mainstream society. Their diversity reflects the rich cultural differences of customs, beliefs, countries of origin, and locations in the United States.

Many non-native-born African Americans live in the United States, and have unique health care and service delivery concerns. To adequately address these issues would go beyond the scope of this discussion, which will focus on aspects specific to native-born African Americans.

DEMOGRAPHICS

African Americans, or blacks, are "individuals who racially define themselves as such or are so defined and treated by socially significant others" (Jackson, 1981) and society. In 1770, there were approximately 757,000 African Americans in the United States; by 1980, there were 26.4 million. In 1988, African Americans made up approximately 12.4 percent of the U.S. population (U.S. Bureau of the Census, 1988). Eighty-five percent live in predominantly urban areas of the North and South (U.S. Bureau of the

Census, 1988). In 1980 there were approximately 4 million African Americans living in rural areas of the United States, making them the largest rural racial minority (U.S. Bureau of the Census, 1984). The majority of African Americans who live in rural areas are in the South (U.S. Bureau of the Census, 1989).

Despite their presence at all socioeconomic levels in the United States, African Americans are disproportionately represented in the lower classes (Durant and Louden, 1986; Hill, 1990; Lefall, 1990). The 1990 census indicated that 32 percent of all African Americans were below the poverty level, as compared with only 11 percent of the white population (U.S. Department of Commerce, 1991). About half of all African Americans born in urban areas are born into poverty (Rodgers, 1990), and about half of these are born to single young adults or teenage parents (Rodgers, 1990).

There is an increasingly negative disparity in mortality rates among African Americans, other people of color, and the U.S. population as a whole (Lefall, 1990). Although 1989 National Center for Health Statistics data indicated that neonatal and postnatal deaths declined similarly for African Americans and whites, the differential gap did not decrease: African Americans still have twice as many pre- and postnatal deaths as whites of the same age (teens to age twenty-four) (Hughes, 1989; Wegman, 1990). The leading causes of death for African Americans are heart disease, cancer, stroke, diabetes, liver disease, asthma, tuberculosis, and, recently, AIDS. The leading causes of premature death—which include smoking, excessive drinking, excessive weight, substance abuse, increased risk of accidents, suicide, and homicide—are significantly influenced by personal behavior and life style. Family disruptions and poor performance at school or work can lead to acute and chronic medical conditions.

RELIGION

Spirituality, in one form or another, plays a major role in the lives of many African Americans. Because beliefs in God or "spirits" and the people in roles of spiritual authority (e.g., ministers) greatly influence the health-care decision-making of many African Americans, it is important for the health professional to have some understanding of the role these beliefs and authorities play in the lives of clients (Kleinman, 1979).

Most African Americans who are religiously oriented are affiliated with a Protestant faith, commonly Baptist (Poole, 1990). The primary mission of the "corporate church" has been to "uplift the masses" by serving as an agent of social control with respect to the family (Poole, 1990). The black church is the most important organization in African American life, serving as the ethical and moral center of the community (Poole, 1990).

Folk medicine and other religious conventions, like voodooism, are practiced in one form or another by native- and non-native-born African Americans alike. Dennis (1979, p. 12) noted that these "unconventional healers" are common in the African American community and are often used in conjunction with "conventional healers," such as physicians. The use of folk medicine and similar practices is based on the individual's belief regarding the etiology of a malady. For example, if an individual believes that he or she is ill because of being out of favor with God or a "spirit," then he or she may seek interceding prayer from a spiritualist (Dennis, 1979).

BELIEFS ABOUT HEALTH

In the African American community, beliefs about health are based on individual and collective experiences as well as on sociocultural norms and education. For example, if a condition does not interfere with activities, it is often considered not serious enough to warrant care. Likewise, if the care for a condition can be administered over a short period of time, this is preferred to care requiring a lengthy protocol. These behaviors have implications for the delivery of genetic services. A main tenet of genetic counseling is the "communication of facts about the disorder in question to couples at risk" (Bowman and Murray, 1990, p. 345), and this communication process stretches over the period of time from the identification of the "at-risk" condition to follow-up after conception (or beyond). For many African American couples, the time required for this degree of involvement is prohibitive.

In general, African Americans have less contact with and use of medical or dental services than do whites (Heckler, 1985). The differences are more pronounced when broken down by age, showing a ratio of 2:1 nonminority to minority children (Heckler, 1985). In addition, minorities are less likely than whites to use preventive health services (Sherzer, Druckman, and Alpert, 1980; Heckler, 1982; Anderson, 1983). From 1978 to 1980, only six of every ten African American women sought prenatal care during the first trimester of pregnancy, compared to eight of ten nonminority women (Anderson, 1983; Heckler, 1985). Despite the 2:1 ratio of low birthweight and postnatal deaths of African Americans to whites as recently as 1989, African Americans continued to use postnatal follow-up services far less than whites. Even when controlling for many of the enabling factors (such as income and medical coverage), the use of genetic and other preventive services by African Americans and other people of color remains limited (Heckler, 1985).

African Americans in the middle class are more able to afford good quality health care and tend to be more consumer oriented than those in the lower class. But despite their class advantage, middle-class African Americans still experience discrimination in the health care system, especially on an interpersonal level. Health care providers tend not to make class distinctions among African Americans, the result being erroneous assumptions about clients' backgrounds and health care experiences that perpetuate stereotypes, miscommunication, and conflicts between practitioner and client.

The literature suggests that the negative past experiences of many urban African Americans with the medical system influence their behavior (Morrill, 1970; McKinlay, 1975; Acton, 1976; Haynes, 1981; Jackson, 1981; Anderson, 1983; Smith, 1987; Friedson, 1988). Some of the experiences reported include the perception of a judgmental attitude by a usually white counselor (90 percent of all masters-level genetic counselors are white [Wiel and Lessing, 1991]) and an impersonal attitude toward addressing the individual's concerns by not explaining more about the diagnosis at the first encounter (McKinlay, 1975; Smith, 1987). As a result, many African Americans fear and distrust the traditional / orthodox health care system. In hemoglobin trait counseling, for example, fear and distrust may be exacerbated by communicating the fact that hemoglobin variations primarily affect people of color.

This lack of trust frequently leads African Americans and other people of color to seek alternative sources of health care. Despite the existence of a formalized system to help families in need (i.e., social workers, psychologists, medical professionals), African Americans are more likely to use informal networks (i.e., family members, folk healers) as a source of information and social support (Jackson, 1981).

Most minorities prefer a network that they perceive as more in tune with their culture than the formalized medical system (Friedson, 1988; Jackson, 1981). Many African Americans are more likely than whites to lack economic resources or insurance to pay for medical services (Rundall and Wheeler, 1979; Anderson, 1983) and, given their economic and racial status, to have experienced discrimination or denial of services (Dixon, 1986). These social barriers lead to an attitude or behavior of presenting medical difficulties "only when they have to" (Suchman, 1966; Stein and Jessop, 1985). African Americans are less likely to view preventive services as "worth the time" and opt instead for resources with a higher potential for success or immediate attention (i.e., folk healers) (Suchman, 1966; Aday, 1975; Jackson, 1981; Sawyer, 1982).

THE DELIVERY OF HEALTH SERVICES

The history of health services to African Americans demonstrates how the legal and health care institutions have reflected society's view of a group of individuals whom the Constitution records as "three-fifths" of a person. Even once slavery ended, a pattern of segregation was enforced. Segregated services for African Americans, with theoretical formulations that distinguished whites from others without regard for culture or class, were widespread until the mid-1960s. Many of these theoretical formulations were based on the premise that African Americans were inferior—a subspecies of human (Thomas and Sillen, 1972).

The formulations resulted in several inaccurate theories:

1. The genetic fallacy, which articulates the genetic inferiority of African Americans
2. The deficit idea, which articulates the theory of cultural deprivation and deficiency
3. The mark of oppression, which proposes that all African Americans are oppressed as a result of slavery and thus tend to return to certain characteristics (the term *oppression* denotes that African Americans are limited or lacking in some irreversible way)
4. The illusion of color blindness, which negates the patient as an individual and a member of any specific group (it is more comfortable not to "see" color, because it negates responsibility for any problems or prejudices regarding color)

Applying cultural, psychological, and sociological characteristics indiscriminately to all members of a particular group risks the danger that services, even when provided, will be affected. It also reinforces a constellation of negative and mistrustful attitudes and beliefs about the medical system in the African American community (Levy, 1985).

Chamberlain (1974) detailed the views held by the majority group toward African Americans, poor people, and other people of color in delivering health services (table 3.1). He argued that these views are based on negative "implied causes," which are stereotypical misconceptions about the social and health practices of African Americans and others that ignore the reality in which these individuals live. As a result of the adoption of these views, he pointed out, even when services exist, there are inherent barriers at individual, institutional, and societal levels. Practitioners must be aware of these views and their potential consequences when devising programs to deliver health care to African Americans and others.

In general, African Americans experience complex health disadvantages that are exacerbated by a combination of poverty, racial bias, ignorance, and lack of access to good quality health care. Although African Americans as a group frequently suffer from discrimination, prejudice, and socioeconomic deprivation, each individual experiences this from a different economic, class, and interpersonal standpoint. This diversity of experience is a key factor in the delivery of preventive and medical services, such as genetic services, to this population (Jackson, 1981).

Murray (1980) suggested that ethnic and cultural backgrounds may influence the way persons approach problems and family members' receptivity to assistance, advice, and guidance. The background differences between the family and the health professional, either individually or in combination, can affect communication, the impact of the disorder, the extent of the support structure, the extent of acceptance in the community, the willingness to seek helpful advice, and the receptivity to different medical actions and interventions. According to Murray (1984), cultural and ethnic differences can be identified and defined to encompass race, religion, sex, and socioeconomic status. To avoid stereotyping, practitioners should use such information as guidelines rather than generalizations (Murray, 1984). Williams (1986) suggested that when socioeducational and economic factors are controlled for, the use of mental health services is the same for whites and African Americans in the middle and upper middle classes. Different authors suggested analogous considerations in the rendering of services to African Americans (Nash, 1986; Davis and Proctor, 1989; Randall-Davis, 1989; Bowman and Murray, 1990). Murray et al. (1980) posited that these considerations include (1) cultural factors, (2) social and educational factors, (3) economic factors, (4) problems of access to diagnostic and therapeutic services, (5) a generalized suspicion and fear of governmental controls and processes, and (6) language difficulties or differences.

Table 3.1. Factors to Consider in Devising the Content of a Health Program for African Americans

Views of the Black Community Found in Health and Sociological Literature	Implied Causes	Reality-Related Views of the Black Community
A higher rate of povety at all times, prosperity or depression, unemployment and underemployment prevalent	Unwillingness to work, desire for welfare	Restricted from open membership in many industries, unions, training programs, businesses, etc.
Overcrowded, inadequate housing poorly maintained, predominantly rental	Lack of standards or interest in improving neighborhood	Fewer options in housing, less access to mortgages for home ownership, higher prices demanded
Inferior educational system	Reduced capacity of students to achieve academically	Inequitable allocation of budget, personnel, equipment, and resources
Non-nuclear, disorganized family unit without strong two-parent heads	Pathological, matriarchal	Extended family concept and need for more than one income to survive
Poor nutritional habits leading to health problems	Ignorance of proper nutritional habits	Reduced income, less access to variety of foods in corner stores, prices in neighborhood consistently higher
Underusage and infrequent use of available community agency resources	Lack of interest	Limited access to information re: resources, negative experience with disrespectful treatment and ineffective treatment
Absence of interest in health education and preventive health measures	Lack of value system for prevention, preference for crisis treatment	Inaccessibility to respectful efforts to communicate re: preventive measures and health education
Overuse of emergency room for ongoing health care	Apathy, ignorance of the importance of health	Insufficient funds for private medical care, limited number of physicians who will accept Medicaid, Medicare, language barriers between non-English-speaking practitioners and native-born blacks
Inconsistent use of health facilities and noncompliance with regimen as given (diet, prescriptions, etc.)	Inability to adhere to a prescribed plan	Lack of communication, inaccessibility of facilities, disrespectful attitudes on part of providers

Table 3.1 (continued)

Resistance to information related to control of family size	Lack of concern and understanding of population crisis and its relationship to quality of life	Knowledge of genocidal and unethical practices, recognition of effect of racism on quality of life

Source: Adapted from Chamberlain (1974)

The American society's ambivalence and uncertainty toward the idea of equality in medicine has generally led to a disregard of ethnic differences and to the perpetuation of the white middle class as the norm. Such prevailing thoughts have socialized health practitioners and health settings and have led to dysfunctional attitudes and behaviors toward those who may be culturally or racially different. Such attitudes have included the denial of any cultural or racial differences, and the superimposing of the Western "culture of medicine" (Friedson, 1988) on the cultural/belief systems of African Americans. Another attitude—fear—stereotypes African Americans as a potentially volatile group. Belief in this stereotype dictates that providers be concerned for their own safety. Another attitude is myopic missionary zeal in helping the downtrodden and oppressed. Disrespectful behaviors can include condescension toward those seeking help, an authoritative reaction to questions, an expression of annoyance to questions about what the provider is saying, a defensive posture, the rejection of a client's interpretation of the problem, and a general lack of meaningful interest.

It is important for the practitioner to take into account the client's level of participation in and commitment to a culture and identity. English (1983) conceptualized a window of four quadrants that define an individual's level of cultural commitment and participation (figure 3.1). This suggests that views of culture and identity are determined by an interaction among the ethnic culture, the mainstream culture, and the individual's critical life events and experiences. Quadrants 1 and 2 represent people with a strong commitment to their own culture and identification with the mainstream culture, while quadrants 3 and 4 represent people with a weak commitment to both their own and the mainstream culture.

One approach to discerning cultural (and racial) nuances is the use of the Cultural Status Exam (Pfefferling, 1981). The exam is composed of six questions (table 3.2), which elucidate information about cultural beliefs and attitudes, health and medical practices, the impact and significance of the family, the degree of adaptation to or assimilation into mainstream Amer-

Figure 3.1.

Level of Participation in and Commitment to One's Own Culture and Identity

		High	*Low*
Level of Participation in and Commitment to Mainstream and Other Cultures	*High*	(1) Bicultural/ Multicultural	(2) Acculturated/ Assimilated
	Low	(3) Native-Oriented/ Traditional	(4) Transitional/ Marginal

Source: Adapted from English (1983)

ica, communication barriers, and attitudes toward health. This exam enables the health service provider to better understand an individual's health belief system and to determine the degree of acculturation to mainstream Western medicine, while beginning to rate the cultural and racial influences that have implications for the delivery of health services.

The use of assessment tools such as the Cultural Status Exam allows health service providers who are aware of cultural and racial differences at least to begin to listen to what a patient might be saying, rather than superimposing their belief system on him or her. Further, it enables providers to reframe their impressions and discuss them in the context of the patient's belief system. Providers can acknowledge differences and make recommendations through an increased understanding of clients' perceptions and how they view their difficulties.

IMPLICATIONS FOR GENETIC SERVICES

Genetic services include medical, educational, and support programs. Effective delivery of genetic services must begin with an understanding of what factors may influence how services are offered and received. The delivery of genetic services to African Americans requires a biopsychosocial perspective. An individual is composed of physical (molecular), cellular (an organ system), and psychological (cognitive, affective, and behavioral) components. The conceptual framework for the delivery of services goes beyond

Table 3.2. Questions in the Cultural Status Exam

1. How would you describe the problem that has brought you to me?
   a. Is there anyone else with you whom I can talk to about your problem? (If yes, to significant other: Can you describe X's problem?)
   b. Has anyone else in your family / friend network helped you with this problem?
2. How long have you had this (these) problem(s)?
   a. Does anyone else whom you know have this problem? (If yes, ask the patient to describe them, how old they are, and the different manifestations.)
3. What do you think is wrong, out of balance, or causing your problem?
   a. Who else do you know with this kind of problem?
   b. Who or what kind of people don't get this problem?
4. Why has this problem happened to you, and why now?
   a. Why has it happened to (the involved party)?
   b. Why are you sick and not someone else?
5. What do you think will help clear up your problem?
   a. (If the patient suggests specific tasks, procedures, or drugs, ask the patient to further define what these are and how they will help.)
6. Apart from me, who else do you think can help get you better?
   a. Are there things that make you feel better or give you relief that doctors (or health care providers) don't know about?

Source: Adapted from Pfefferling (1981)

the components and examines the person as part of a larger interacting and interdependent unit with numerous influences, including social, cultural, racial, geographical, and economical, as well as those of medical care and the general physical environment (Dilworth-Anderson et al., 1994).

Randall-Davis (1989) proposed a useful conceptualization for offering genetic services to African Americans, which includes a clinical application of specific cultural values. Incorporated with the health belief system (Kleinman, 1979; Harwood, 1981), this gives a useful perspective in rendering medical services. The conceptualization must be in relation to a determination of the degree of acculturation to the mainstream Western notion of medicine and socioeconomic class services. The sophistication in medical assessment and diagnosis is absent in the consideration of race, ethnicity, and class issues (*New York Times,* 25 September 1990).

Several investigators have pointed to the significance of race and ethnicity in relation to genetic conditions. Vichinsky (1980, 1983) suggested that patients with sickle cell disease might avert the complications of transfusion if they receive blood donated by African Americans. Bowman and

Murray (1990) said that genetics should have at least equal weight with environmental factors in determining health. A *New York Times* article (25 September 1990) reported: "Genetics is playing a predominate role in that it determines a predisposition to conditions produced by the environment. . . . Environment can trigger the expression of genetic disease and if it were not for social and economic factors, many genetic diseases would stay dormant and people would never suffer from them."

The literature addressing the compliance of African Americans and other people of color in newborn screening is scarce (Jackson, 1981; Smith, 1987). However, the literature on the use of pre- and postnatal preventive services by African Americans and others (Anonymous, 1972; Jackson, 1981; Bowman, 1983; Scott, 1983; Whitten and Nishiura, 1985; Smith, 1987; Pachter, 1989) suggests that many psychosociological factors contribute to this limited use of counseling services. For example, Jackson (1981, p. 68), in discussing the relationship between low birthweight and lack of prenatal care among African Americans, pointed to individual, social, and structural factors that may hinder the delivery of preventive and trait follow-up services:

> Among many lower-class (African American) women, a major deterrent to prenatal care has been a prevailing belief that the natural function of childbearing requires no medical intervention until the delivery stage. But even among those who may have desired care, other problems deterred them, including inadequate funds, lack of access, difficulty in arranging medical visits, and the "forbidding settings and brusqueness" of some maternity clinics. Moreover, many unwed mothers attempted to conceal pregnancies as long as possible.

Since a majority of individuals with hemoglobinopathies are people of color—a recent study found rates of 1:8 African Americans, 1:10 Asian Americans, and 1:50 Hispanic Americans, compared to 1:125 for whites (Vichinsky et al., 1983)—providers disseminating genetic information should be sensitive to issues of these populations, particularly since the majority of the providers are white (Weil and Lessing, 1991). Practitioners may choose to point out the genetic advantage of sickle trait (protection from malaria) when conveying this information to patients. This stresses the positive rather than the negative aspect of genetic alterations.

The turbulent events surrounding sickle cell testing programs serve as an example of the larger issue of the ability of African Americans and other people of color to understand, gain access to, and use preventive medical services offered by the orthodox medical system (Nash, 1983, 1986). Roland B. Scott, of Howard University, and colleagues were instrumental in influencing Congress to pass the National Sickle Cell Anemia Control Act in 1972 (Scott, 1983). Before this, sickle cell trait and disease had received very little national attention. The 1972 act allowed for "the establishment of comprehensive sickle cell centers, screening and education clinics, a mission-oriented research and development program, biomedical research, an educational program, and a hemoglobinopathy detection training program" (Scott, 1983). This act brought hope that through national legislation a condition affecting one of every four hundred African Americans would receive the attention needed to combat its adverse biological, psychological, and social consequences.

But, as Dr. Scott (1983, p. 349) pointed out, "the path from obscurity to prominence was cluttered with many unfortunate circumstances and complaints." Mass screening for sickle cell trait and disease in the early 1970s was in many cases a political and social disaster. Confusion, fear, and widespread discrimination against trait carriers were evident. For example, people with the trait were denied health insurance and life insurance and many were dismissed from their jobs (Scott, 1983; Whitten and Nishiura, 1985) despite overwhelming evidence that sickle cell trait is not associated with adverse medical problems (Vichinsky, Hurst, and Lubin, 1983; Edelstein, 1986; Gaston, 1987). Other unfortunate circumstances included: (1) the regarding of mass screening by some as a means to further shame and degrade African Americans, (2) encouragement by many African American leaders to avoid screening because of the possible adverse effects of job loss and insurance denial, and (3) the push of well-meaning legislators to enact policies that would require sickle cell testing either on entering school or as part of premarital testing. This precedent created a lack of interest in and trust of sickle cell screening programs by both public officials and people at large and led to an unfavorable attitude about testing that has begun to wane only in recent years (Bowman, 1983; Whethers, Pearson, and Gaston, 1989). A clear message of these events is that the process involving the dissemination of vital information that will potentially affect the livelihood of others should be well thought out, evaluated, and relevant to the population it is intended to reach.

Other barriers to the genetic counseling process include practical circumstances that make it difficult for African Americans to receive counseling. For instance, many families have working parents who are unable to take time off during the day to receive counseling. Limited means of transportation creates difficulty when traveling to counseling centers that are far away. Urban African Americans and other people of color are more likely to use community and medical services that are both financially and physically accessible and that are known to be available when they need it (Jackson, 1981). This accounts for the higher use of emergency room and public clinics as primary sources of care by urban African Americans than by their white counterparts (Aday, 1975; Andersen and Aday, 1978; Telfair, 1983).

The experiences of many African Americans who must use public facilities for medical care often involve a long time in the waiting room, traveling some distance to receive care, receiving fragmented care, and, because most public facilities are teaching facilities, possibly seeing a different physician at each visit (Stein and Jessop, 1985). These structural barriers serve to reinforce negative attitudes toward seeking care (Langlie, 1977), which further contribute to a lower use of services as well as the client's fear that an extra effort must be made for preventive follow-up counseling (Gochman, 1972; Aday, 1975).

The delivery of genetic services to African Americans living in rural areas poses a unique challenge due to the prevailing lack of, and limited access to, orthodox social and health services (Farley, 1988; Rounds, 1988). Because social networks and local healers have traditionally provided many of these services under the sanction of the religious community, it is important for practitioners to involve local healers in the process of delivering information and services.

In the delivery of prenatal and postnatal care, the practitioner needs to take a comprehensive approach to include other health and environmental risk factors (e.g., diabetes, poverty). The practitioner should also consider new paradigms for the delivery of services, such as developing a collaborative relationship between the health care provider and the patient. This helps to empower clients and allows them to intervene in some of the social interferences that affect their care. For example, clients can help develop more effective treatment services by giving their feedback on the timing of visits to the clinic for therapy or counseling (e.g., after work or school on certain days of the week).

To best understand the individuals presenting themselves for services, providers must understand the important cultural values and behaviors of their clients, as well as the incidence of genetic disease (see table 3.3). Cultural universals include family relations, health beliefs, religious beliefs and their interrelationship with health beliefs, sexual attitudes and practices, drug usage / habits, and styles of communication.

Table 3.3. Genetic Variations and Disorders More Commonly Found in African Americans

Anthropometry and Skeletal Variations
  Stature
  Birthweight
  Growth
  Body size and form
  Teeth and jaw abnormalities
  Hand abnormalities
  Brachydactyly type D
  Carpal fusion anomalies
  Joint hypermobility
  Variation in number of vertebrae
  Anterior femoral curvature
Normal and Abnormal Pigmentation
  Differences in melanosomes
  Oculocutaneous albinism
  Ocular albinism
Dermatoglyphics
  Distal phalanges
  Special palmer formulations
  Down syndrome dermatoglyphics
Polymorphic Variation
  Chromosomal variation
  XX true hermaphroditism
  Blood group polymorphisms (ABO most studied)
  Enzyme polymorphisms
  Hereditary elliptocytosis
  Serum protein polymorphisms
  HLA polymorphisms
  DNA polymorphisms
Glucose-6-Phosphate Dehydrogenase Deficiency (G-6-PD)
Hemoglobinopathies and Thalassemias
  Sickle hemoglobinopathies
  Alpha thalassemias
  Beta thalassemias
  Globin gene polymorphisms
Lactose Intolerance and Malabsorption
Twin and Other Multiple Births
Congenital Malformations
  Musculoskeletal malformations
  Polydactyly
  Taipes equinovarus
  Hip malformations

Table 3.3 (continued)

Central nervous system malformations
α-Fetoprotein and neural tube defects
Cleft lip, cleft palate, and cleft gum
Ear malformations
Hypoplasia of the lung
Cardiovascular malformations
Supernumerary nipples
Small bowel atresia
Down syndrome

Source: Data from Bowman and Murray (1990)

RELIGION

It is important for a practitioner to determine the client's religion (if any) and the attitude toward science and medicine espoused by that religion, and then to work within the individual's belief system. If it seems appropriate, providers should involve the church or the minister in the treatment plan. The minister is an important influence in the Christian community. He or she usually knows the emotional and psychological makeup of the parishioners. Religion also affects many African Americans' beliefs about illness and health. For example, many emotional problems are seen as punishment for disobeying God or as the devil's work. It is important to emphasize that the individual has the ability to help God's plan. Providers should be aware that guilt may influence a client's perception of illness. Helping clients identify causes of illness and specific actions they can take not only supports their values and beliefs but also enhances the practitioner-client relationship.

Folk medicine often exists alongside biomedicine in both the determination of and the remedy for a particular illness. Practitioners should ask clients if they believe the illness was caused by any other means, such as being hexed. Providers should ask them and the involved family members and / or advisers whether the involvement of folk healers would be helpful in this situation. African Americans will often use herbal and home remedies, seek spiritual advisers, wear charms and other objects for protection against evil spirits, or engage in other rituals of healing. It is not uncommon for there to be beliefs about blood, hot and cold, the role of drafts in illness, religiously based illness, and psychosomatic causation.

Other illnesses are believed to be caused by witchcraft or possession by evil spirits, particularly in lower socioeconomic groups and rural groups. Common terms for witchcraft or the possession of evil spirits include *fixed, mojoed, hooded, hexed,* and *rooted.* For example, "crazy" behavior or seizures are thought to be signs that the person is rooted. These episodes are usually related to both internal and external stress. The practitioner should be aware that the person receiving genetic services will almost never volunteer the information that he or she has been hexed, but usually will respond to direct questions if asked in a nonjudgmental fashion.

Practitioners should always convey a nonjudgmental attitude toward whatever method of treatment the client and / or family has tried already or is currently using. If practices do not endanger the client's health, providers should leave them alone, and try to incorporate treatment suggestions into this ongoing system by emphasizing the natural origins of medications and treatments that derive from naturally occurring substances.

Individuals of African descent are diverse, and as unique as their mixed ancestry. Therefore, attitudes toward the use of DNA storage, autopsy, family planning, amniocentesis, chorionic villus sampling, and artificial insemination will vary according to religious and cultural beliefs. These procedures may also be viewed as irrelevant, particularly if the financial situation is precarious; access is limited or difficult; comprehension of science is limited; or the family holds fatalistic beliefs.

FAMILY

Extended family and kinship networks are important to African Americans. Members are counted on for moral support, financial aid, and help in crisis. Generally there is a flexibility of roles within the family, so decision-making may rest with either the male or the female head of the household. For African Americans, the involvement of the extended family in the treatment process is important. The provider must determine who the significant decision-maker is and involve that person in the treatment plan. Family structure may include actual and fictive kin, who may or may not have shared authority in decision-making. It is important to have some understanding of the structure and roles of all members and to use this knowledge in the counseling / interview session(s).

Elderly members of the community are respected. Providers should address elderly African Americans by title and last name, and consider involving elderly persons in the treatment process, particularly the grandmother, if she is highly visible. Individuals coming in for genetic services may have first consulted the "mother-adviser" on the block.

Maternal wisdom is a valued commodity in the African American community. Often it is the mother's responsibility to identify problems and decide what to do. Seeking professional consultation depends on the perceived severity of the condition by the mother (or mother figure) and the belief that treatment will cure the problem. Practitioners should involve the mother or mother figure in treatment, and address concerns regarding treatment to the mother and the patient.

Many adults, be they fictive or actual kin, are important in child-rearing and influential in the shaping of youth. When working with children, providers should involve these significant adults in the treatment process. These roles are valued; reliance on these individuals by young adults remains an important aspect of their decision-making process.

Children are socialized to keep cool under pressure and learn survival skills from their elders. One of the skills is not to reveal true feelings, so it is important for the physician / counselor to encourage the expression of feelings of stress as a means of ascertaining factors influencing the well-being of African Americans and the effective provision of health services.

Adoption outside the family may not be well accepted. Families take care of "their own" and frown upon giving up a child. Nonpaternity does occur, and anecdotal evidence suggests higher incidence in families of lower socioeconomic levels. However, practitioners should use caution in discussing this subject; preservation of the family unit, as it exists, is very important. Consanguinity is taboo, as in the larger North American culture.

COMMUNICATION

It is not uncommon for African Americans to look at someone when they are talking and to look away while listening. Prolonged eye contact is considered staring and may be unacceptable. While conversing, they may engage in other activities, such as nodding the head and making responses to indicate listening (Randall-Davis, 1989). Also, African Americans tend to move closer than whites when talking. They tend to display an attentive affect when speaking, but less when listening, and are usually quick to respond. The communication style is more affective, emotional, and interpersonal (Sue and Sue, 1990). Depending on social class, age, educational, and economic factors, African Americans may use nonstandard English language, that is, the jargon and slang indigenous to a subgroup. Examples can be found in rap and hip-hop music and talking "jive."

It is critical to understand these cultural differences so as not to misinterpret them. Practitioners who are not sure of what is being said or do not understand the variation of the language that may be used should so indicate or ask for elaboration before making a decision. Understanding these differences and allowing the client to define the perimeters of the contact is important. This requires a reconsideration of the standardized notion of how help should be given by different professional disciplines.

The Perception of Time

According to their social class and degree of acculturation, African Americans tend to be present oriented and not preoccupied with the future. Historically, providers have viewed this orientation as a hindrance to the dissemination of knowledge about pre- and postnatal care (and other preventive care). There may exist, then, two competing agendas. For example, many African Americans may not understand why a follow-up meeting designed to explain a diagnosis is needed if this explanation can be given at the time of diagnosis; what they really want to know is what they are supposed to do to deal with the condition now (Haynes, 1981). On the other hand, practitioners view the follow-up counseling as an essential step in the diagnosis and treatment of an anomaly (Costello, 1987).

In working with African Americans, practitioners should foster a focus on the immediate situation rather than on future plans. Once the immediate situation is handled, there can be a discussion of the concept of prevention of chronic complications and long-term plans. For example, in delivering genetic counseling to parents who seem more concerned with housing or food, the counselor should work to help the client meet these instrumental needs before attempting to deliver genetic information.

Counseling

Illness, particularly mental illness, can be seen as caused by disturbance in interpersonal relations, demonic possession, or brain injury. Receiving help for such conditions is often seen as a stigma and as threatening. In counseling African Americans, practitioners should ask patients what they believe is the cause of the problem, and emphasize the importance of seeking professional help for stress or other troubles. African Americans frequently do not self-refer to agencies specializing in counseling and mental health services. Their presence in such an agency indicates that problems are advanced and the individuals are at high risk. It is important to create an atmosphere in which the practitioner gives the individual permission to have problems. A calm exterior or nonverbalization of stress does not necessarily indicate that there is none.

African Americans have come to rely on their own resources and take care of their own problems. There may be a reluctance to discuss family problems and personal relationships with outsiders. They may downplay the severity of their problems and indicate that they have the situation under control when, in fact, they do not. It is not uncommon for African Americans, when seeking help out of necessity, to focus on survival issues rather than psychological needs. Practitioners should acknowledge the individuals' priorities, and help them to meet their basic needs. This may mean referral to other agencies that can assist with instrumental needs such as housing, food, or financial and legal services. Counseling services might well be accepted as appropriate.

Middle-class and urban African Americans are more likely to use counseling or mental health agencies for emotional problems than lower-class and rural African Americans, who are more likely to rely on family members, ministers, or physicians for these problems. Many African Americans use both the formal mental health system and the informal community system for health and mental health problems. Knowledge of these patterns of service use can often prove useful in designing strategies for long-term intervention. It is imperative to provide immediate and specific solutions and advice with respect to the client's problems. It may be necessary to refer the individual to another treatment facility or to work in collaboration with a minister or other identified helper. It may also be necessary for persons rendering the counseling services to reveal something about themselves, to establish rapport and trust.

CONCLUSION

To minimize the differences between the health care provider and the African American client, both the provider and the institution must commit to the creation of a climate of cultural diversity. This begins by building a culturally diverse staff, developing a culturally diverse administration, generating financial support for training for diversity, creating a support system, developing a multicultural perspective in the client care program, and preparing for the consequences of change.

So often, work is focused on the practitioner and not the institution. With institutional commitment, serious attempts can minimize the differences, which would include reexamining the client-practitioner relationship and the role expectations of both, recognizing the power relationship and gender differences, accepting the client's perception of service, responding to client needs, and coping with culturally valued differences within the context of the ethnic and racial backgrounds of both the client and the practitioner. This will facilitate managing discrepancies that may exist, through client / staff education, working within the patient's conceptual system, and negotiating a compromise.

SUMMARY

—Greet and address individuals formally. Do not use first names unless requested.

—Do not imitate jargon; this may be perceived as ridicule.

—Assess the patient's educational level and address concerns accordingly.

—Involve community leaders and patients in establishing clinics and clinic hours.

—Be aware that because of the "fiasco" with mass sickle cell screening, males may be especially reluctant to admit they are carriers. They may also be unwilling to accept information about positive carrier status.

—When imparting knowledge about sickle trait, stress the positive: the genetic advantage regarding malaria.

—Keep eye contact while engaged in discussion, but avoid staring.

—At the first session, explain the counseling session, follow-up, etc. Give suggestions related to the present. The future can be addressed at a later time.

—Family support systems may be more important than those outside the extended family.

—Utilize the Cultural Status Exam before the counseling session.

—Assess the issues of the community being served (financial problems, access to care, etc.). Try to hold clinics at convenient times and accessible locations.

ACKNOWLEDGMENTS

This research was supported in part by grant PH60HL28391-06 from the National Heart, Lung and Blood Institute to the second author.

We thank Michelle Hughes for her critical comments and editing on earlier drafts of this manuscript.

REFERENCES

Acton, J. P. 1976. Demand for health care among the urban poor with special emphasis on the role of time. In Rossett, R. N. (ed.), *The Role of Health Economics in the Health Service Sector,* pp. 165–214. New York: New York Bureau of Economic Research.

Aday, L. A. 1975. Economic and noneconomic barriers to the use of needed medical services. *Medical Care* 13:447–56.

Andersen, R., and Aday, L. A. 1978. Access to medical care in the U.S.: Realized and potential. *Medical Care* 16:533–46.

Anderson, J. R. 1983. The black experience with the health services delivery system. In Johnson, A. E. (ed.), *The Black Experience: Considerations for Health and Human Services.* Davis, Calif.: International Dialogue Press.

Anonymous. 1972. Ethical and social issues in screening for genetic diseases. *New England Journal of Medicine* 286:1129–32.

Bowman, J. E. 1983. Is a national program to prevent sickle cell disease possible? *American Journal of Pediatric Hematology / Oncology* 5:367–72.

Bowman, J. E., and Murray, R. F. 1990. *Genetic Variation and Disorders in Peoples of African Origin.* Baltimore: Johns Hopkins University Press.

Chamberlain, N. 1974. Sickle cell anemia: Community education programs in black communities. In Murray, R. (ed.), *Handbook for Genetic Counseling in Hemoglobinopathies.* Washington, D.C.: Howard University Center for Sickle Cell Disease.

Costello, A. 1987. Psychosocial management of patients in a fetal medicine and surgery program. *Birth Defects* 23:62–74.

Davis, L. E., and Proctor, E. K. 1989. *Race, Gender, and Class.* Englewood Cliffs, N.J.: Prentice Hall.

Dennis, R. E. 1979. Health beliefs and practices of ethnic and religious groups. In Watkins, E. L., and Johnson, A. E. (eds.), *Removing Cultural and Ethnic Barriers to Health Care: Based on Proceedings of a National Conference,* pp. 12–28. U.S. Department of Health, Education, and Welfare. Washington, D.C.: GPO.

Dilworth-Anderson, P., Harris, L. H., Holbrook, C. T., Konrad, R., Kramer, K. D., Nash, K. B., and Phillips, G. 1994. Graphical representations of biopsychosocial models of health and illness. *Journal of Health and Social Policy* 5:185–202.

Dixon, M. A. 1986. Families of adolescent clients and non-clients: Their environments and help-seeking behavior. *Advances in Nursing Science* 8:75–88.

Durant, T. J., Jr., and Louden, J. S. 1986. The black middle class in America: Historical and contemporary perspectives. *Phylon* 47:253–63.

Edelstein, S. J. 1986. *The Sickled Cell: From Myth to Molecules.* Cambridge: Harvard University Press.

English, R. A. 1983. *The Challenge for Mental Health Minorities and Their World View.* Austin: University of Texas Press.

Farley, E. S. 1988. Cultural diversity in health care: The education of future practitioners. In Van Horne, W. A., and Tonnesen, T. V. (eds.), *Ethnicity and Health.* Milwaukee: University of Wisconsin Press.

Friedson, E. 1988. *Profession of Medicine: A Study of the Sociology of Applied Knowledge.* Chicago: University of Chicago Press.

Gaston, M. H. 1987. Sickle cell disease: An overview. *Seminars in Roentgenology* 22:150–59.

Gochman, D. S. 1972. The organizing role of motivation in health beliefs and intentions. *Journal of Health and Social Behavior* 13:285–93.

Gorman, C. 1991. Why do blacks die young? *Time,* 16 September, pp. 50–52.

Harwood, A. 1981. *Ethnicity and Medical Care.* Cambridge: Harvard University Press.

Haynes, A. 1981. The gap in health status between black and white Americans. In Hayes, W. A. (ed.), *Health Status and Health Delivery Systems and the Minority Community: A Reader,* pp. 1–30. Berkeley: University of California Press.

Heckler, M. M. 1982. *Health of Minorities and Women.* U.S. Department of Health and Human Services. Washington, D.C.: GPO.

————. 1985. *Report of the Secretary's Task Force on Black and Minority Health.* U.S. Department of Health and Human Services. Washington, D.C.: GPO.

Hill, R. B. 1990. Economic forces, structural discrimination, and black family instability. In Cheatham, H. E., and Stewart, J. B. (eds.), *Black Families: Interdisciplinary Perspectives,* pp. 87–105. New Brunswick, N.J.: Transaction Publishers.

Hughes, D. 1989. The health of America's children: Maternal and child health data book. Washington, D.C.: Children's Defense Fund.

Jackson, J. J. 1981. Urban black Americans. In Harwood, A. (ed.), *Ethnicity and Medical Care.* Cambridge: Harvard University Press.

Kleinman, A. 1979. *Patients and Healers in the Context of Culture: An Exploration of the Borderland between Anthropology, Medicine, and Psychiatry.* Berkeley: University of California Press.

Langlie, J. K. 1977. Social networks, health behavior, and preventive health behavior. *Journal of Health and Social Behavior* 18:244 60.

Lefall, L. S. 1990. Health status of black Americans. In Dewart, J. (ed.), *State of Black America,* p. 121. New York: Transaction Publications.

Levy, D. R. 1985. White doctors and black patients: Influence of race on the doctor-patient relationship. *Pediatrics* 75:639–43.

McKinlay, J. B. 1975. The help-seeking behavior of the poor. In Kosa, J., and Zola, I. K. (eds.), *Poverty and Health: A Sociological Analysis,* rev. ed., pp. 224–73. Cambridge: Harvard University Press.

Morrill, D. L. 1970. Factors affecting distance traveled to hospitals. *Economic Geography* 46:161.

Murray, R. F., Jr. 1984. Cultural and ethnic influences on the genetic counselling process. In Weiss, J. O., Bernhardt, B. A., and Paul, N. W. (eds.), *Genetic Disorders and Birth Defects in Families and Society: Toward Interdisciplinary Understanding,* pp. 71–74. White Plains, N.Y.: March of Dimes Birth Defects Foundation.

Murray, R. F., Jr., Chamberlain, N., Fletcher, J., Hopkins, E., Jackson, R., King, P. A., and Powledge, T. M. 1980. Special considerations for minority participation in prenatal diagnosis. *Journal of the American Medical Association* 243:1254–56.

Nash, K. B. 1983. Overview of humanistic progress in sickle cell anemia during the past ten years. *American Journal of Pediatric Hematology/Oncology* 5:352–59.

————. 1986. Ethnicity, race, and the health care delivery system. In Hurtig, A. L., and Viera, C. T. (eds.), *Sickle Cell Disease: Psychological and Psychosocial Issues.* Urbana: University of Illinois Press.

Pachter, L. M. 1989. Cultural considerations in pediatrics. In Schwartz, M. W., et al. (eds.),

Pediatric Primary Care: A Problem-Oriented Approach, 2d ed., pp. 11–16. Chicago: Year-book Medical Publishers.

Pfefferling, J. H. 1981. A cultural prescription for medicocentrism. In Eisenberg, L., and Kleinman, A. (eds.), *The Relevance of Social Science to Medicine,* pp. 197–222. Boston: D. Rendel.

Poole, T. G. 1990. Black families and the black church: A sociohistorical perspective. In Cheatham, H. E., and Stewart, J. B. (eds.), *Black Families: Interdisciplinary Perspectives,* p. 3349. New Brunswick, N.J.: Transaction Publishers.

Randall-Davis, E. 1989. *Strategies for Working with Culturally Diverse Communities and Clients.* Washington, D.C.: Association for the Care of Children's Health.

Rodgers, H. J., Jr. 1990. *Poor Women, Poor Families: The Economic Plight of America's Female-Headed Households.* Armonk, N.Y.: M. E. Sharpe.

Rounds, K. A. 1988. AIDS in rural areas: Challenges to providing care. *Social Work* 33:257–61.

Rundall, T. G., and Wheeler, J. R. C. 1979. The effect of income on use of preventive care: An evaluation of alternative explanations. *Journal of Health and Social Behavior* 20:397–406.

Sawyer, D. O. 1982. Assessing access constraints on system equity: Source of care differences in the distribution of medical services. *Health Services Research* 17:27–44.

Scherzer, L. N., Druckman, R., and Alpert, J. J. 1980. Care-seeking patterns of families using a municipal hospital emergency room. *Medical Care* 18:289–96.

Scott, R. B. 1983. Historical review of legislative and national initiatives for sickle cell disease. *American Journal of Pediatric Hematology/Oncology* 5:346–51.

Smith, S. C. 1987. Barriers to cross-cultural counseling: The American black perspective. *Birth Defects* 23:183–87.

Stein, R. E. K., and Jessop, D. J. 1985. Delivery of care to inner-city children with chronic conditions. In Hobbs, N., and Perrin, J. M. (eds.), *Issues in the Care of Children with Chronic Illness,* pp. 382–401. San Francisco: Jossey-Bass.

Suchman, E. A. 1966. Health orientation and medical care. *American Journal of Public Health* 56:97–105.

Sue, D. W., and Sue, D. 1990. *Counseling the Culturally Different.* New York: John Wiley & Sons.

Telfair, J. 1983. Utilization of a public hospital's "walk-in" clinic: An examination of three variables. Master's thesis, University of California, Berkeley, School of Public Health.

Thomas, A., and Sillen, S. 1972. *Racism and Psychiatry.* New York: Brunner/Mazell.

U.S. Bureau of the Census. 1984. Urban and rural populations by race. In *Statistical Abstract of the United States, 1985,* 105th ed. Washington, D.C.: GPO.

———. 1986. *Vital and Health Statistics: Use of Selected Preventive Care Procedures, United States, 1982.* Data from the National Health Survey, ser. 10, no. 157. Washington, D.C.: GPO.

———. 1988. Components of population change. In *Statistical Abstract of the United States, 1989,* 109th ed. Washington, D.C.: GPO.

U.S. Department of Commerce. 1991. *Poverty in the United States, 1990,* Current Population Reports (Consumer Income), ser. P-60, no. 175. Washington, D.C.: GPO.

Vichinsky, E. P., and Lubin, B. H. 1980. Sickle cell anemia and related hemoglobinopathies. *Pediatric Clinics of North America* 27:429–47.

Vichinsky, E. P., Hurst, D., and Lubin, B. H. 1983. Sickle cell disease: Basic concepts. *Hospital Medicine* 19:128–58.

Wegman, M. E. 1990. Annual summary of vital statistics, 1989. *Pediatrics* 86:835–47.

Weil, J., and Lessing, S. 1991. Personal communication.

Whethers, D., Pearson, H., and Gaston, M. 1989. Newborn screening for sickle cell disease and other hemoglobinopathies. *Pediatrics* 83:813–914.

Whitten, C. F., and Nishiura, E. N. 1985. Sickle cell anemia. In Hobbs, N., and Perrin, J. M. (eds.), *Issues in the Care of Children with Chronic Illness,* pp. 236–60. San Francisco: Jossey-Bass.

Williams, D. H. 1986. The epidemiology of mental illness in Afro-Americans. *Hospital and Community Psychiatry* 37:42–49.

4

Culture of Native Americans of the Southwest

*Lynn Hauck, M.A., M.S., and
Ursula M. Knoki-Wilson, C.N.M., M.S.N.*

There are more than forty tribes of Native Americans across the southwestern United States. This chapter will focus on the Pueblo tribes of Hopi and Zuni, and the Athapaskan tribes of Navajo and Apache.

HISTORY

Pueblo, the Spanish word for "town," refers to the village-dwelling Indians of the Southwest. There are approximately fifteen pueblos across Arizona and New Mexico. Pueblos were founded near a spring or other source of running water, which encouraged an agricultural life style. The Hopi of northeastern Arizona and the Zuni of New Mexico are Pueblo Indians. Both groups are believed to be descended from the prehistoric Anasazi peoples. There are ruins in an abandoned Hopi village which date back to A.D. 1150, and abandoned pueblos in Canyon de Chelly date back to A.D. 700. The Hopi language is a Shoshonean dialect of the Uto-Aztecan linguistic family (Waters, 1977), while the Zuni language has roots in the Zunian linguistic branch (Dozier, 1970).

Some time before A.D. 1500, the hunting and gathering Athapaskan tribes came into the Southwest from the north and east. These immigrants are known today as the Navajo and the several Apache bands. The Navajo and Apache are part of the southern division of the Athapaskan linguistic stock. The Athapaskan groups form the most widely dispersed linguistic family in North America; parts of this family can be found not only in the Southwest but also in Alaska, Canada, and the Northwest Coast, the last representing the earliest known homeland of the group after they crossed the land bridge from Asia (Melody, 1977). Initially a patrilineal society with patrilocal residence, the Athapaskans are believed to have had a "shamanistic, individual religion preoccupied with curing" (Hester, 1962).

Once in the Southwest, the Navajo went through a series of cultural changes in adapting to the natural environment, which was vastly different from that of the north, as well as adapting to social contact with the established Pueblo peoples. As they recognized the advantages of the Pueblo culture, they began to adopt practices beneficial to them. They developed a horticultural life style, raising corn and maize (Leighton, 1966).

The Apache were far more migratory than the Navajo. The Apache, a hunting and fighting people, preferred mountainous terrain, traveling from ridge to ridge with the weather and the food supply. They were not organized into any tribal political unit, preferring instead small groups of bands. "The band was the political unit, with leader and followers. This system did not have a tribal chief, no council of leaders and exercised no control over a specific portion of the land" (Basehart, 1970). Bands grew, lost members, and disappeared, and new groups developed.

The term *Apache* comes from the Zuni word for "enemy," *A'pachu* (Melody, 1977); in fact, the Apache refer to themselves as the *N'de, Inde, Tinde,* or *Dini,* which translates simply as "the people." The Apache are divided into six regional groups. The more plainslike, eastern Apache include the Jicarilla, Kiowa, and Lipum. The more westerly Apache include the Mescalero, Chiricahua, and Western Apache. The Western Apache were the most sedentary, as they depended the most on agriculture. The clan relationships among the Western Apache were initially related to where a band had a right to grow food in a season (Haley, 1981).

The Pueblo societies were well established when Coronado's expeditions arrived in the 1540s. In their drive to increase landholdings, the Spanish settlers moved northward from Mexico and over the next century took possession of Pueblo country. They gave Pueblo settlements the names of Spanish saints and divided the land area into districts, assigning a Catholic priest to each. Oaths of obedience as well as deference to the Catholic Church and the Spanish crown were expected of the pueblo inhabitants (Dutton, 1975). The increasing numbers of Spanish people edged into desirable Pueblo holdings. They attacked the pueblos frequently, burning structures and killing or capturing individuals.

Encouraging a return to traditional religion and culture, Pope, a Pueblo medicine man, led a revolt against the Spanish. In August 1680, he and his followers killed approximately four hundred Spanish missionaries and colonists; others were pushed southward to El Paso. They then destroyed Christian churches and other evidence of Spanish occupation (Folsom, 1973). In 1692, two years after Pope's death, the Spanish returned. To resist the Spanish threat, the Hopi built permanent settlements atop the three high mesas they occupy today. The Zuni also used elevation to their advantage, and retreated to Corn Mountain. As a result, the Spanish were unable to return with any force.

The Navajo and Pueblo peoples came together to ward off the Spanish and provide temporary homelands for the Pueblo refugees. "In a space of a few years, the Navajo adopted Pueblo styles of architectural, manufacturing techniques and religious paraphernalia plus many elements of non-material culture such as clans, matrilineal descent, matrilocal residence, the origin myth and ritual" (Hester, 1962). These changes did not affect the preference for the hogan, a type of house that can be traced to Asia, as their place of residence. "Pueblo and Navajo ceremonial items have been excavated from the same creches, giving credence to the belief that much modern Navajo ceremonialism is derived from the early Pueblo contacts. Pueblo influences including sand paintings, metate and fire pit styles and weaving, at least in part, altered the basic Navajo culture, and within a few centuries distinguished it from that of the Apache who had less contact with the Pueblo people" (Dutton, 1975). The Spanish had brought horses, sheep, and goats as well as silversmithing, which were adopted by both the Pueblo and the Navajo peoples.

From the 1600s on, the Navajo persistently raided the villages of their Pueblo neighbors as well as those of the Spanish and, later, Mexican colonists. The migratory life style of the Apache precluded occupation by the Spanish. By 1688, most of the Apache groups were supplementing their agricultural and hunting activities with raids on the Spanish and western-migrating Anglo settlers. Navajo raids were particularly devastating to the western pueblos and to Mexican and Anglo holdings during the middle of the nineteenth century.

Spanish rule ended with the Mexican Revolution of 1821, after which the Mexican government declared that Native Americans were citizens on an equal basis with all others. Mexican rule did not significantly change life for Native Americans. The Mexican-American War ended with the Treaty of Guadalupe Hildalgo in 1848. In this treaty the United States gained all land east of the Rio Grande as well as the land areas of modern-day New Mexico, Arizona, Utah, Nevada, and northern California for the price of $15 million. Articles of the treaty indicated that the U.S. government was to recognize and protect Native American rights previously established under Spanish and Mexican rule.

When the United States gained possession of the Southwest, many land treaties were made and broken due to communication difficulties and lack of enforcement on the part of the U.S. government. In 1863 James Carlton assigned Kit Carson to round up the Navajo and Apache peoples and convince them to become sedentary agriculturists like their Pueblo neighbors. Men, women, and children were rounded up across Navajo territory. Livestock and food supplies were destroyed, and those individuals who refused to come were killed. The Athapaskan people were held at Fort Sumner, New Mexico, for four years.

This attempt at "taming" the people was a failure. Crops that the Navajo and Apache were forced to plant did not thrive due to insects and drought. The crowded camps bred discontent, disease, and a great number of deaths. When the impracticality in both monetary and human expense became apparent, a treaty was concluded in August 1868, establishing a 3.5-million-acre reservation, a small portion of their former holdings. At this time, the tribe numbered around nine thousand. The Treaty of Bosque Redondo promised clothing, goods, raw materials, sheep, and cattle to the Navajo. The quantity, quality, and timing of delivery of these goods were inadequate, and most of those who returned from Fort Sumner subsisted on the berries, nuts, and grains they could gather and the game they could kill.

Reservations had been established in all of the pueblos by 1890. Some of the boundaries were based on the former Spanish land grants, while others were established by the U.S. government. The Navajo (Dene, the Navajo Nation) have had several land disputes with the U.S. government. The original 3.5 million acres was increased periodically to the nearly 14.5 million acres that they now hold (Dutton, 1975). The Hopi reservation is surrounded by Navajo land, and disputes over these boundaries continue today. The Apache occupy reservations in Arizona, New Mexico, and Oklahoma.

Hopi

Hopi means "peace." All thought, word, and deed is dedicated to maintaining harmony through the actions of the self, the community, and the universe; this is the "Hopi Way." Three interrelated forces in Hopi life are the clan, the household, and the religious society (Thompson and Joseph, 1944).

A clan is made up of several families. The members of the families are related through the mothers (matrilineal descent) and take the mothers' clan name. The name and function of the family are not as important as the clan to which they belong. The clan determines an individual's standing in religious and secular matters. Certain clans are more important than others by reason of the offices or ceremonies they control. The important clans have a ritual or ceremony whose power benefits all the community. Currently, the Bear Clan is at the top of the hierarchy. Each clan has the name of an animal, bird, or other living entity, and each has a special guardian spirit symbolized by a wood or stone fetish. A clan pharity is a group of related clans that share a fetish. If the Bear Clan is the ancestral clan, related clans in this pharity are the Black Bear, Gray Bear, Strap, Grease Eye Socket, Bluebird, Mole, and Water Coyote. There are approximately twelve major clans and twenty-nine subclans.

The clan chiefs are determined through the female line: a man's sister's son succeeds him into office. The leaders of the various clans comprise the council. The village chief of Oraibi, the center of Hopi ceremonial life, is the head of the Bear Clan. He directs council activities and has the right to veto proposals brought before the council. In Hopi theory, the village chief owns in trust all the land around the pueblo, all the houses, and all the crops. If disputes arise concerning land or property, he has the final word in settling them. The crier chief, head of the Reed Clan, has the responsibility of announcing upcoming ceremonies and public functions as well as the decisions of the council (Waters, 1977).

There are many small villages across the three widely separated mesas, which were founded by different clans. Because each clan has its own secrets and ceremonies, it is impossible for one individual or one clan to hold all of the secrets and all of the power. When disputes arise within a clan, the peace-loving Hopi Way encourages a split of the clan, with some of the members relocating and often renaming themselves. This clan system does not lend itself to unity or centralization, and the Hopi have never viewed themselves as a tribal whole. There is no central government or supreme chief.

The household or group of households is a unit of central significance within the clan. This unit is composed of a woman, her daughters, her granddaughters, any unmarried sons of these women, and the husbands of married women. Thus, the household consists of a group of closely related women who have grown up and worked together in the same family. The women own the home, the small garden adjoining the home, seed for the next year's planting, as well as the springs and cisterns. The men do the farming away from the village as well as finding and hauling fuel; traditionally, men did the skinning, weaving, and moccasin-making. Even though a man lives in the household of his wife, on ceremonial days and during other activities relating to his clan family, an association with his mother's and sister's homes continues. He also serves as the chief disciplinarian and source of punishment for his sister's children. A Hopi baby is a *member* of the mother's clan and a *child* of the father's clan. The same distinction holds for one's mother, mother's sister, maternal grandmother's sister's daughter, and all members of the clan whom one's mother calls "sister." Within the clan, the children of all the women called "mother" are one's brothers and sisters (Aberle, 1951). There are cultural taboos against marrying into the father's clan or within a clan pharity. Before marriage, the female will approach her grandmother to ask whether a blood relationship exists between the family of the husband-to-be and her own.

If an individual has not been married before, tradition dictates that he or she should not marry a divorced or widowed person, or else the journey to the underworld afterlife will be affected. Adolescent sex is tolerated, and only if the couple is getting too involved and the girl's parents disapprove of her choice do her parents interfere. Nonpaternity does not appear to be problematic. Marriages tend to become more stable after children are born. Young children stay with their mother, and older children have a choice of living with either parent. It is believed that unfaithfulness and fighting will bring illness to and perhaps even the death of a young child (Aberle, 1951). Common reasons for separation include a violent temper, laziness, stinginess, or adultery. Divorce can result from the wish of either partner.

Another important component of Hopi culture is the religious societies to which men and women belong. When a child reaches the age of six to ten, he or she is initiated into the *kachina* cult. This introduces individuals to "their ancestors, the kachinas." A version of the kachina legend relates that the kachinas were gods who used to come when the people were sad or lonely. They danced and taught hunting, industries, and arts. As the people began farming, the kachinas would dance in the fields when rain was needed. When the people began to take these benevolent beings for granted, they decided to leave. But before they left, they taught the dances to a few loyal followers and instructed them in making masks and costumes. As long as the instructions were followed and their "hearts were right," the people were allowed to act as kachinas and the real kachinas would come and possess the person acting the part of the kachina. Rain would come.

The kachina mask unites people and spirit beings. The kachina cult exists for the purpose of impersonating the supernatural rainmakers, so that weather controls may be exercised and moisture for the crops and pasture will result. The Pueblo feel that they are an important part of nature, that all parts of the universe are interrelated, and that they and the universe must be kept in balance. If this equilibrium is upset by selfish or hostile attitudes, disaster will result. Each person considers it his or her duty to perform ceremonies to help the seasons follow one another in proper succession, to promote the fertility of plants and animals, to encourage rain, and to ensure successful hunting. All this is voiced in prayers and dramatized in dances (Dutton, 1975). When the kachina cult functions fully, every man, woman, and child of the pueblo is initiated into it, and every man takes part in the ceremonies. Upon death, a Pueblo person becomes a kachina and may appear as ancestors in the form of a cloud.

As part of the preparation for a child's initiation into the kachina cult, the biological parents select ceremonial parents to sponsor and help guide the child. The ceremonial parents must belong to a different clan from either biological parent, and when the child is an adult, he or she is expected to join one or more of the secret societies of the ceremonial parents. Each society has a secret initiation and certain dances and ceremonies, as well as specific healing ceremonies (Thompson and Joseph, 1944). For example, the Lakon Society, which is a women's society, is said to possess the power to heal skin trouble by using a particular plant. Lakon belongs to the Badger Clan, and the badger is an animal that knows all plants. Each society is thought to cause as well as cure a specific disease or ailment. Some individual medicine people use simple remedies and herbs to cure minor ailments. The members of the important societies deal with major afflictions. Each great clan has a certain time of year when its special ceremony is performed. The only hope of help from the gods is felt to come through these powerful priesthoods. The control of rainfall and the harvest as well as causing and curing disease are ceremonials controlled by the priesthoods. A sick person applies to the society for a cure. A specific ceremony may be performed or the disease may be drawn or "sucked out." A separate ceremony to envision the cause of the disease is not required (Underhill, 1965). It is believed that disease can be caused by the individual's failure to pray, perform ritual activities, or exhibit correct conduct, which helps to maintain the universe in a harmonious state, particularly with regard to rainfall, the growth of crops, the movement of the sun and moon, and human reproduction.

Zuni

The Hopi and Zuni have many similarities in culture and religion, but the Spanish influence surfaces in the religious practices of the Zuni more than in those of the Hopi. The Zuni religion incorporated Spanish beliefs in death rituals, such as the washing of the body, the all-night vigil, and wailing women (Parsons, 1916). The Catholic Church's influence manifests itself in the observance of All Souls' Day, when the children sing a Latin-derived song as they go from house to house, as well as in the parading of the Santo during the harvest dance in the fall (Parsons, 1917).

Navajo

Navajo culture is matrilineal. The Navajo grandmother is the center of the home. The children belong to her and are members of her clan. To look upon or talk to one's mother-in-law is taboo. The daughter and her husband live in a separate hogan, so the daughter and the children go back and forth between the dwellings. Several generations may live in close proximity to one another. The women own and care for the home, livestock, and crops. Property ownership is individual. A woman sells the rug she weaves, the crops she cultivates, and the stock she cares for, and spends the money earned as she pleases. A man does likewise with the silver jewelry he makes, the wages he earns, and the profits from his livestock or farming. The man represents the family in public and at ceremonials. Marriages are allowed after clanships have been determined. One of the major cultural differences between Pueblo and Athapaskan is that the Pueblo value the group as a whole and an individual's contribution to the group, while the Navajo consider the individual the most important.

The Navajo ceremonials, in contrast with those of the Pueblo people, do not place emphasis on weather control, and in particular rain-making. Navajo religion centers on curing ceremonies in which harmony is restored. All rituals are performed with a specific aim in mind, such as ensuring survival, restoring health, or securing food.

> In the Navajo universe, two classes of personal forces are recognized, human beings and the holy people or supernatural beings; holy in that they are powerful and mysterious. The Navajo believes his universe functions according to certain set rules. If one learns these rules and lives in accordance with them, he will keep safe or be restored to safety. The supernatural beings have great power over those on earth, but they can be coerced and supplicated by man. . . . The universe as viewed by the Navajo is an orderly system of interrelated elements, an all inclusive unity that contains both good and evil. Therefore, the universe is good, benevolent and dangerous. With the Navajo concept of the universe being in a state in which good and evil are maintained in interrelated harmony, the problem is in maintaining that harmony [Dutton, 1975].

The primary purpose of the ceremonials, called "sings," is to keep humankind in harmony with the universe. The ceremonials are conducted by a singer or chanter. Most singers know two or three complete ceremonials and specialize in those; it would be impossible for one person to learn all the complicated rituals for more than a few ceremonials. In a ceremony called the Night Way, there are at least 576 songs, and each must be word-perfect and uttered in perfect intonation to accomplish its purpose. In addition to memorizing all the songs for a ceremony that may go on for nine days, the healer must also hold in mind the details of the symbols and their positions, the equipment, and the elaborate rituals and dances, and must direct the creation of dry paintings (Kluckhohn, 1962). Ceremonies involve time and many people and can be very costly to the family.

If universal harmony is disturbed, it is believed that illness, death, or other disaster may occur. Tradition holds that illness has supernatural causes and may be traced to some transgression on the part of the victim. Disease, misfortune, distress, and other evil caused by failure to observe taboos and ceremonial regulations by spirits, by natural elements, or by phenomena such as whirlwinds, lightning, water, or, worst of all, witchcraft, are reasons for a ceremonial. Each rite is especially adapted to a particular set of uses and to combat or thwart one or another disease or misfortune. The specific ceremony required is determined by divination, itself a ceremony carried out by a process of hand-trembling, stargazing, or listening. A diviner interprets the involuntary motions of his hands or things he sees or hears while in a trancelike state, and discovers the cause of the trouble. He determines the proper ritual for cure and may recommend a singer.

The curing chant ways are always concerned with a specific disease. The Hail Way and Water Way treat illness resulting from cold or rain. The Shooting Chant is used to cure injuries received from lightning, arrows, or snakes. Snakes are also an important factor in the Navajo Wind Way and the Beauty Way. The Beauty Way is used against aching feet, legs, arms, back, and waist, as well as swollen ankles. Itching skin, mental confusion, insanity, and paralysis require the Night Chant (Haile, 1938).

Among most Native Americans of the Southwest, the dry painting plays an important part in the curing ceremonies, but no other peoples have developed this art to the degree that the Navajo have. There are between six hundred and one thousand separate designs; there are thirty-five different dry paintings for the Red Ant Way ceremony alone. Most often the singer directs the "painters" but does not directly participate in the creation of the paintings. The painting is created on sand or sometimes on cloth or buckskin with the use of coarse sand, cornmeal, flower pollen, powdered roots, stone, and bark. Because of the sacred nature of the ceremony, the paintings are begun, finished, used, and destroyed within a twelve-hour period. The purpose of the painting is curative; it is believed that by sitting on the representations of the holy people in the dry painting, the patient will become identified with the holy people and absorb some of their power (Locke, 1989).

The Navajo greatly fear death and everything connected with it. This intense feeling stems from the fear of ghosts and witches of the afterworld. They fear that the dead may return as ghosts to plague the living. Therefore, any dead person is considered a potential danger. Ghosts are believed to take the form of human beings, animals, birds, whirlwinds, spots of fire, and other items. They appear only after dark or at the approach of a death. Ghosts may foreshadow general disaster as well as harm to an individual. When a Navajo sees a ghost or dreams of one, it is imperative that the proper ceremony be performed or else the individual will surely die. If successful, such ceremonial cures are believed to have killed the witch one way or another (Dutton, 1975).

Apache

The Western Apache adopted matrilineal descent and matrilocal residences. The home structure was a modified tepee called a *wickiup* (Dutton, 1975). When a daughter married, her mother and sisters would construct a new wickiup near the mother's home.

As mentioned, clans began as a group of individuals allowed to grow crops in a particular area. These groups evolved into a second kind of family, apart from blood relations, who would help in revenge raids and other family-like activities. Sixty clans have been identified, taking their names from a unique feature of the clan or a physical feature at or near the farming plot.

The head man was chosen because of admirable personality traits, and the head woman consulted on the ways of living and led food-gathering activities. Personal honor and honesty were key elements in a good life. A broken promise would bring swift and mighty revenge (Dutton, 1975).

Marriage was not allowed within a clan or between the relatives of one's mother's or father's clan. Each clan was considered to be closely related to a few others and marriage between certain clans was also prohibited. However, marriage was allowed within the same band (Goodwin, 1942). (The clan system cuts across bands and groups.) Chastity was highly regarded and a virgin bride brought more gifts from the prospective groom's family than a bride who had been sexually active. A marriage could be forced if it was found out that a couple had had intercourse.

Today, certain relationships remain strong. Apache mothers and daughters are very close and perform many tasks together. When a son marries, his obligations are to protect and work for the domestic circle into which he marries. Divorce can be requested by either member of the couple, and usually involves consultation with the wife's family. Divorce is usually discouraged; however, it would never be prohibited. Reasons for divorce include incompatibility, laziness, and infertility.

The Apache prize children highly and usually space them four years apart. Babies and toddlers are indulged and their care is shared by all women in the household. When the child is about six to twelve months old, a *di yan* or shaman performs a hair-cutting ceremony. The hair is cut close to the scalp, leaving a couple of long strands. The shorn hair is then buried under a fruit tree, often with a piece of the di yan's hair. This ceremony is performed every year for four years. After that the hair is never cut, to avoid bad luck. Other ceremonies for children include the first moccasin ceremony, some time between nine months and two years of age, to put the child on the Apache life way or path. Coming-of-age ceremonies are held for males and females. The four-day ceremony for young women is better known than the ceremonies for young men.

Healing ceremonies are usually held for individuals by a shaman who has specialized in a particular area of healing. Any person may become a shaman. A vision or dream may signify special talents in healing. A child may become a shaman for a time and lose the talent as he or she grows older. An individual who is interested in learning the chants and secrets held by a particular shaman approaches the shaman with a gift. If accepted, the individual and shaman live together until the novice has learned the dances, chants, and prayers.

BELIEFS ABOUT HEALTH

The Native American beliefs stated here are generalizations; they are not universal for all tribes or for any one tribe. Several factors that influence beliefs are: the amount of time and the experiences a person has off the reservation, formal education, influences of an outside religion intertwined with clan or subtribe affiliation, membership in a tribal society, and marriage. Health care providers should never assume that an individual knows traditional beliefs or identifies with them.

Among the majority of Native American cultures, there is a high degree of integration between religious beliefs and beliefs about health. Neither social behavior nor healing can be separated from culture, sacred narratives, or religion (Levy, 1974). The Navajo have no distinct term for religion. The healing ceremonies are an integral part of the community experience (Kluckhohn and Leighton, 1962). Aberle (1966) was unable to discern a difference in traditional healing and religious practices of Native Americans. There is little difference between a church and a hospital or between religion and medicine. The Native American belief system considers health a spiritual as well as physical state.

Native Americans believe in the Supreme Creator, who is an all-powerful spiritual being. The Supreme Creator is never impersonated in tribal rituals and ceremonies. There may be a specific name for this individual, which is often regarded as sacred, including the Hopi "Original Being," the Navajo "First Being," or the Apache "Giver of Life." The Supreme Creator is often accompanied by spirit beings, which may be a partner, mate, cocreator, or offspring of the Supreme Creator. These lesser individuals are often represented in ceremonies. The spirit beings are held responsible for both the good fortune and the bad luck that befall humans. An example of these spirit beings are the Navajo monster slayers, which are the twin offspring of Navajo deities.

Many cultures recognize spirit helpers, who are similar to angels and saints in the Euro-American culture. They command thanks and respect but are not gods and are not the object of prayer. The Hopi have kachinas, the Navajo have Yei, and the Apache have the Ghan or Mountain Spirits. By donning masks and other ceremonial garb, a dancer invites the spirit helper to inhabit his or her body. This brings insight, knowledge, and spiritual blessings to the group. (Compare this to single individuals such as a minister or priest in other organized religion. The spirit of God is invited through the priest to bless the congregation. The evangelist's prophecy is to speak in tongues and heal as a "host" of the Holy Ghost.) In many Native American cultures, healing rituals are performed by a group rather than by an individual. The Hopi kachina dancers may number as many as a dozen, and each individual dancer is responsible for a "vital component which contributes to a complete, harmonious ceremony" (Locust, 1985b). The Apache female coming-of-age ceremony involves the young woman's becoming the incarnate Changing Woman, a female deity with special powers. She is accompanied by five or more Ghan (Mountain Spirit) dancers, who bring blessings to the tribe (Locust, 1985a).

Native Americans believe that the individual is made up of mind, body, and spirit. The Hopi song to welcome a newborn baby into the world invites a "spirit" to inhabit the body that the parents have created. An Apache medicine person identified this spirit as "the one who I am." A number of Native American groups, including the Laguna, Seneca, and Comanche, view the body as an instrument through which the spirit may express itself, become aware of spiritual lessons, and progress toward the ultimate goal of being united with the Supreme Creator.

It is believed that the physical body contains the spirit or Supreme Identity; the mind links the body and the spirit. An individual may hear a truth with his or her ears, the spiritual component of the individual recognizes this truth, and the mind translates this truth by making adjustments in the consciousness to utilize this new truth. Once this adjustment or manipulation has taken place, harmony has occurred among the individual, the Supreme Creator, the environment, and the universe.

Vitality through creation is usually referred to as power. This energy or power is spiritual in nature. It can be manifest through an individual (such as a healer or medicine person), a stone (such as a crystal, which may have healing powers), or a plant (which may be powerful for its curative or sedative properties). A medicine person is one who knows which objects, plants, stones, or other materials contain various powers and how to use these powers. The treatment of disease among many Native American groups incorporates the basic tenet of the threefold composition of body, mind, and spirit. Contemporary Western medicine may view that a "cure" has taken place after the surgical repair of a congenital cardiac defect. The Navajo family may feel that only the symptoms have been treated and that the underlying cause of the heart defect is spiritual in nature and, thus, the spirit must also be treated. Often the individual or family may desire to consult with a medicine person or participate in a healing ceremony as well as utilize Western medicine. The medicine person restores harmony among mind, body, and spirit; the Western physician heals the body.

A strong Native American belief holds that the spirit world is intertwined throughout all of nature. All things have a spirit, and the spirit part must be recognized and honored. When an ear of corn is harvested, the corn plant should be thanked for giving of itself. After killing an animal, a hunter may give a gift in return, maintaining harmony in both the physical and the spiritual worlds. A plant imparts both physical and spiritual healing properties: the physical in the form of stems, leaves, and roots; the spiritual essence in the curative properties of the plant as it relieves suffering. Prayer and ceremony may also be directed toward inanimate objects and natural phenomena. A carver may thank the tree from which the wood came. A potter may sing to the spirit in the clay as he or she forms the pots.

Many animals and birds can appear in spirit form without a physical body. Dreams and visions involving specific animals are regarded as very important. The adolescent coming-of-age ceremony or "vision quest" may involve the vision of an animal from the spirit world becoming the symbol for his or her life. Spirits without physical forms are considered part of a world parallel to the physical world, existing side by side within the physical world but also intermingling with it. Medicine people often "see" into the spirit world, either in the present or in a continuum of time. Many Native Americans are aware of the spirit world and regard it as a natural element of existence.

Belief in immortality among Native Americans incorporates a belief in an existence as a spiritual being before physical life begins as well as a return to a spiritual life with the Supreme Creator. The belief that a spiritual identity coexists with the physical identity enables the spirit, once the physical body is dead, to return to the spirit world and then arrange to go back to the physical realm. The Pueblo people believe that when a baby dies, the spirit will return in the next baby born to the same parents. After an umbilical cord dries up and falls off, it is attached to an arrow and placed beside a beam overhead in the main living room. This would house the spirit of the baby in the event of death. The spirit would await the opportunity to return in the body of the next child conceived (Talayesva, 1942).

The circular and continuous nature of existence obviates any belief in final judgment or divine retribution (Hultkrantz, 1979). The tribe identifies where a spirit continues its existence in various physical states, including where it rests, repents for past deeds, or progresses into spiritual understanding. Spirits who are visiting the earth can be seen in dreams and visions. Communication from these individuals is regarded as highly significant. Medicine people may foretell who they will be when they return. A child might tell of events in a previous life.

The interaction of the mind, body, and spirit is at the core of Native American traditional healing. When people feel either physically or psychologically ill, they explore why they have brought themselves to this event. Setting and casting a broken arm quickly remedies the physical aspects, but the underlying spiritual causes of the event must also be sought. Once identified, an individual can begin to change that aspect of his or her body, mind, or spirit that was out of harmony. Sometimes a medicine person must be consulted to aid the individual in understanding the relationship among mind, body, and spirit. Rehabilitation therapy, antibiotics, prostheses, crutches, or wheelchairs assist the affected body. Ceremonies, signs, herbs, prayers, and rituals assist the affected mind and spirit. Wellness is achieved when there is harmony among mind, body, and spirit. Harmony refers to a state of "oneness" with the self, life, eternity, and the Supreme Creator.

Harmony is established when the individual becomes conscious of why he or she is on earth as well as of the personal relationship with the Supreme Creator. Once this difficult and elusive relationship is established and incorporated within the self and the surrounding environment, the person feels anchored to Mother Earth. This may be associated with the adolescent coming-of-age ceremonies. Once this internalization has taken place, the spiritual part of the individual can establish harmony with the Supreme Creator. Wellness or harmony is the same for all individuals; however, the components for any individual may differ. As opposed to achieving perfection, nirvana, or euphoria, achieving harmony is really an attitude about life, and this attitude creates personal peace. Each individual has unique life events with which to deal; for one it may be failing vision, for another pain associated with an injury. The attitude with which one deals with these events is key in maintaining harmony. By making choices, each individual is able to control the maintenance of spiritual connectedness even when he or she cannot control the events of the outside world.

If wellness is synonymous with harmony, then unwellness is equivalent to disharmony in either the body, the mind, or the spirit. Disharmony in one area will affect the others. When one aspect of an individual is out of harmony, the complete individual is unwell. Disharmony of the mind, such as being worried or troubled, does not occur independently, and headaches, insomnia, or ulcers may be the body's manifestation of this unwellness. There is a physical price to pay when an individual has lived for years with the disharmony of suppressed anger, frustration, heartache, or fear.

The causes of unwellness are usually divided into the natural and the unnatural. It is believed that natural unwellness results from a violation of the taboo. This breaking of a strict cultural rule can be done intentionally or unintentionally and can affect the offender or his or her family. Each tribe has identified a certain set of taboos that may be cultural, moral, or religious. Almost every tribe has identified certain creatures, such as insects, spiders, certain reptiles, birds, or other animals, that cause illness or carry negative energy.

The bear has a lot of evil potential for the Apache people; being near a bear or near the place where a bear has eaten or urinated could cause illness (Opler, 1965; Locust, 1985a). The Hopi have stringent rules regarding the care and handling of the kachina masks. Misfortune and illness are bound to befall the violator and may affect his or her family as well. Improper personal conduct may result in a moral taboo. Laughing at a disabled animal or causing a disability in an animal could result in that same disability in an unborn child (Gifford, 1940). A religious taboo would relate to the proper observances of rituals.

Prevalent taboos among many tribes concern death, incest, menstruation, natural phenomena (such as lightning or an eclipse), specific foods or animals, and witchcraft. Menstrual bleeding may be considered unclean or associated with negative energy: a woman who is in her "moon time" must be careful where she goes, what she does, and how she disposes of her sanitary waste. Dire circumstances may follow any deviation from proper behavior.

Unnatural wellness is thought to be caused by witchcraft. Evil is a real and powerful adversary for almost all tribes, and one must be constantly vigilant to guard against it to protect oneself and loved ones. Evil is considered a power and can also be identified as an entity, either human or animal. In any form, evil brings disharmony and can be manipulated by witchcraft. The group of individuals who choose to walk not in harmony but in the power of malevolent spirits and harm other humans are referred to as witches—people skilled in the use of negative power—and their activities are called witchcraft. The concept of witch is not associated with ghosts and goblins but does involve an individual who has performed witchcraft. Witching is manifest in one of two ways: either the environment around the victim is disturbed in such a way as to cause hardship or the individual may be affected directly, resulting in physical unwellness. Among the Apache, the most prevalent kind of witching is "love witching," in which an individual is overwhelmed with the sudden desire to be near a certain person. Many instances of sudden onset, such as accidents, sharp pains, or acute illness, are felt to be related to witchcraft. Anyone who is perceived as predicting the future would also be regarded suspiciously.

Most Native Americans believe in the power of thought and telepathy, whereby a person can affect the emotions and actions of another. A Hopi may believe that each person must be aware of his or her thoughts and words. Negative thoughts or words are like "poisoned arrows that can pierce the heart." Unplanned use of negative energy can be harmful, but the planned, concentrated, and conjured negative power put out by a professional witch can be extremely destructive. This energy is harmful not only to the individual but also to members of his or her family.

If an individual believes that he or she is a victim of witchcraft, then disharmony has occurred. Disharmony allows for spiritual weakness and resultant vulnerability to negative energy. If possible, the individual restores harmony to himself or herself, thereby warding off the negative energy— the spell of the witch. If the individual cannot overcome the spell, then the help of a medicine person may be required. Severe physical illness, depression, or confusion may require a family member to seek the help of a medicine person. The home, immediate family members, and close relatives may be included in the treatment.

Patients must have enough strong spiritual energy to protect their children from negative energy. Lack of spiritual power leads to a, person's violating taboos, which further weakens his or her spiritual power, making the individual and his or her family more vulnerable to both natural and unnatural unwellness.

Many Native Americans hold each individual responsible for his or her own wellness. Wellness and illness are within the control of the individual. When an individual allows himself or herself to become upset, disharmony occurs, resulting, for example, in a headache or other internal discomfort. "Harmony" is a state of being completely attuned to the self, the environment, and the universe. When this state of harmony is complete, moral, religious, or cultural taboos do not occur, nor can negative energy from witchcraft find a weakness to work through. This protective shield is described in a song by the Navajo: "Beauty is above me, beauty is before me, beauty is all around me." Keeping this shield strong affects the individual and tribal well-being.

IMPLICATIONS FOR GENETIC SERVICES

Most tribes consider the responsibility for one's own health to begin before birth, when the spirit chooses the body it will occupy. They believe that others cannot be blamed for the shortcomings of the body because, for whatever reason, we have chosen who and what we are. The spirit knows and accepts the challenges of the physical body. A disabled body is chosen deliberately, with the life's mission in mind. The body may be regarded as disabled but the spirit inside is as strong and wise as the spirit in a normal body.

All cultures have persons with disabilities, but providers must look closely to find out which disabilities are considered handicaps. Confusion may occur when a health care professional attempts to discuss a disability with an individual whose language and culture do not contain such a concept. For example, Lukon interviewed a sister of an elderly Hopi woman who was born with severe kyphoscoliosis. The sister described the woman as "small" and having "a lot of pain in her legs and back." No mention was made of her deformity, and the flavor of conversation was that this "condition" was like a chronic illness that kept her from normal activities. She had status in the community because of her excellent ability to make *piki,* a thin wafer bread (P. Lukon, personal communication, 1985).

There is very little information about Native Americans' treatment of disability. In anthropological descriptions, such names as "red eyes," "little man," "no eyes," "one arm," "big head," and "one who walks with a limp" certainly connote disabilities (Schmitt and Brown, 1968; Brown, 1970). There may be a lack of information on Native Americans' attitudes toward disability because of their reluctance to discuss such personal matters with anyone, particularly non–Native Americans. The intensely personal nature of beliefs, philosophies, and religion is believed to affect past, present, and future lives. The cause-and-effect explanation for life events makes the guilt and fear associated with birth defects obvious. A tribal custom may prohibit talking about such things, to avoid retaliation from other tribal members. Some tribes believe that speaking about a deformity may give it the power to manifest itself in human form. Another reason for the lack of information may relate to the concept that mental, physical, or emotional abnormalities are considered a disease or unwellness, not a disability. For example, some tribes may consider "crazy" people as being special to the gods, not a liability to the tribal community. These individuals may be given specific places in religious ceremonies in the belief that spirits will speak through them (Hultkrantz, 1979). In other tribes albinos hold a special niche (Morgan, 1982).

Tribes differ in what they consider "unwell." The Hopi people view alcoholism not as being unwell, but as a personal choice. They do, however, consider homosexuality a state of unwellness. The Apache people, on the other hand, consider alcoholism, but not homosexuality, as being unwell. Consider the areas of mental retardation, emotional disturbance, or learning disability, which are Western terms implying unwellness. The Native American community may not consider an individual with one of these conditions unwell at all. These individuals may be described as incomplete or slow, but not unwell. The Western preoccupation with labeling conditions often does not translate into Native American languages.

For many groups, the concept of disability may revolve around the ability to perform household tasks, reproduce children, and live a long life. The traditional Navajo family may refuse surgery for congenital hip dislocation if informed that their child may not be able to ride a horse afterward, which, even in today's modern society, is integral to daily life. This quality of "unwellness" may range from a diffuse sense of unrest to the acute pain of arthritis. It may indicate disharmony in the home, on the job, in the environment, or with life.

Besides being aware of the aforementioned concepts and beliefs, health care providers should recognize other important considerations. In greeting families, it is appropriate to address the maternal grandmother first. Providers should use only as much eye contact as is comfortable for the person. Navajos and others may not answer questions immediately, since it is polite and correct to think before speaking. Providers should not interrupt the silence or interpret it as a loss of attention.

The careful history that most tribes maintain about lineage is manifested in strict taboos regarding marriage. To marry within the clan is the same as marriage to a brother or a sister. The result of incest can be seizures, insanity, or "moth sickness." In some tribes it would be considered a great insult to be asked about being related to one's spouse. Rather than ask whether a couple is related, providers taking family histories should inquire as to which clan each person belongs. Remember, individuals may refer to each other as sister or brother when they are not related by blood, but in a ceremonial way. Infertile couples adopt within the tribe, and the line will be matrilineal: the couple adopts a sister's or a cousin's child.

Artificial insemination by a donor is not well accepted, but it should be mentioned as an option in a counseling session. In vitro fertilization and GIFT might be more acceptable if using the couple's own sperm and egg. Diagnostic tests such as venipuncture, skin biopsies, and specimen sample usually present no problems. Amniocentesis or chorionic villus sampling may not be a problem, but since prenatal care is usually sought at a later point in pregnancy, it may not be possible. However, in some cases there may be an opportunity to incorporate both Native American and Western beliefs. A procedure may be more acceptable if the physician's hands are blessed by a native healer before the procedure. Abortion is not taboo, but Down syndrome is not considered a reason for termination. Family planning (birth control, rhythm, etc.) is viewed as an individual choice, but artificial methods are not frequently used. The acceptance of carrier testing is not known. To date, no reasons have compelled using it on a large sector of the population.

In disclosing "bad news" to the family, providers should consider relating it as a story. For example, "Another couple we knew were in a similar situation and this occurred. This is no reflection on your family or ancestors." Physical comfort or touching will probably not be appropriate. Grief is handled quietly or with the family, not in front of strangers. This privacy may extend beyond the living. Most tribes have restrictions about touching the dead, cleansing rituals for those who have had to prepare the body for burial or cremation, and strict procedures about the disposal of property of the dead.

Native Americans may blend Western and traditional medicine as they deal with their own health care. The following case illustrates one family's solution. An Apache child was born with a club foot. The parents allowed him to be sent to an area hospital for corrective surgery. When he returned to the reservation, a healing ceremony was held for him. The family believed that the club foot was caused by the father having cut down a tree for firewood that had been struck by lightning. To the Apache, anything struck by lightning is taboo. If the father had been in complete harmony, he would have known the tree had been struck by lightning and would not have touched it. But being in disharmony, he was unaware of the danger of the lightning spirit. In cutting down the tree, they believed, the man put himself and his family in danger and caused the child to be born with a club foot. A medicine person with "lightning power" performed a healing ceremony to remove the spell that would cause continuing harm to the family. The family believed that the child was not restored to wholeness through either a lack of power on the part of the medicine person or a reluctance to undo what the spirits had done and, perhaps, bring harm upon himself (Locust, 1974).

Biological visual aids can help during the discussion of genetic problems. However, if an individual raises an objection to or rejects the biological theory, the provider should probe the reason for rejection. Sometimes an appropriate ceremony for curing can incorporate Western medical beliefs into Native American healing / health systems.

Native Americans' health care problems include significant consumption of alcohol and exposure to solvent fumes. These have led to high incidence of fetal alcohol syndrome and fetal alcohol effects as well as problems associated with exposure to solvents. However, providers tend to overdiagnose the above syndromes and dismiss other problems of genetic significance. It is well known that the Native Alaskan Yupik Eskimos have a high incidence of congenital adrenal hyperplasia, but there is a significant incidence among the Southwestern tribes as well. Albinism and ichthyosis are also more common, and the disorder Navajo neuropathy does not occur in other groups.

Western medicine is oriented toward fixing a problem, whereas Native American healing works toward developing an individual's power to overcome the illness himself or herself. Traditional medicine people do not heal anyone; they assist individuals in healing themselves. Healing is not synonymous with curing in Native American medicine. A person may never be cured of cancer, but healing can occur if coping occurs on physical, mental, and spiritual levels. Table 4.1 displays some of the conflicting cultural values of the Anglo-American middle class and traditional Native Americans, and draws some lessons for genetic professionals.

CONCLUSION

Native Americans have received poor health service in the past, and their long history of broken treaties has increased their suspicion of Anglos.

Table 4.1. Conflicts in Cultural Values, and Lessons for Genetic Professionals

Anglo-American Middle-Class Values	Native American Traditional Values	Lessons for Genetic Professionals
Mastery over nature: control, subjugate, and overcome	Harmony with nature: be compatible, maintain natural state	Most genetic professionals have been trained in a Western medical model that involves physically and emotionally "fixing" as much as can be "fixed" in any encounter. Be aware that these services are but one resource for the family.
Scheduled living	Nonscheduled living	Making clinic appointments by the clock is unrealistic in a geographically isolated clinic. The reality of the situation may be morning clinic and afternoon clinic. Local ceremonies and weather conditions may make show rates low. Do not be discouraged.
Future oriented	Present oriented	Talking about the outcome of physical therapies, wearing a hearing aid, or participating in Headstart may need reinforcement and encouragement. Be aware in discussions about the future that someone who predicts the future may be regarded as a witch. Instead, work in a storytelling mode. Describe a family with similar life circumstances; tell about the life that that child grew into. Contrast with a family who did things differently. Keep in mind what the local culture regards as a disability. Try to avoid sentences like, "If you do / do not do this, then this will / will not happen."
Competitive, individualism. Always win first place	Noncompetitive, deference to group needs. Win once; let others win	Regard the service you provide as what it is: a consultation. As much as possible, find ways to blend Western medicine and Native American culture. Avoid prejudging individuals, educational levels, or motives.
Acceptance of others on the basis of role and status	Acceptance of others on the basis of demonstrated personal integrity	If materials or services are promised, be dedicated to following through.
Punishment is related to guilt	Punishment is related to shame	No comment

Table 4.1 (continued)

Anglo-American Middle-Class Values	Native American Traditional Values	Lessons for Genetic Professionals
Representative democracy	Face-to-face government; traditionally, little tribal leadership	No comment
Individuality, fame, recognition	Anonymity and humility	Belonging to the group is important. When taking photographs, carefully explain how and where the photographs will be used. Telling a family they might be presented in a paper or at a national meeting may not get an enthusiastic response.
Cultural aspiration to achieve at a level higher than parents; climb the ladder of success	Cultural aspiration to follow in the ways of the old people	Keep in mind the feeling about elders in the group. The elder in the community may be the senior female member. She may or may not be the historian, but impressions and requests may need to be directed to her.
Save for the future	Share resources and wealth with those who need it today	No comment.

Health care providers must realize the family is highly respected and allow the family's involvement in counseling as requested. If the provider is not of the patient's culture, persons who are knowledgeable about beliefs and values should be included.

SUMMARY

—The term *disability* may have different meaning in the Native American culture. Individuals have a place in the society and must be able to function.

—Mental retardation may not be seen as a handicap, since the affected person may be able to plant, make jewelry, and serve other functions.

—Abortion is not taboo, but Down syndrome is not considered a reason for termination.

—Amniocentesis or chorionic villus sampling may not be a problem, but since prenatal care is not sought until a later point in pregnancy, it is a moot point.

—Prenatal procedures may be more acceptable if the physician's hands are blessed by a native healer before the procedure.

—Adoption for infertile couples occurs within the tribe, along matrilineal lines, with the couple adopting a sister's or a cousin's child.

—Artificial insemination by a donor is not well accepted, but it should be mentioned as an option in a counseling session.

—In vitro fertilization and GIFT might be more acceptable if utilizing the couple's own sperm and egg.

—Diagnostic tests such as venipuncture, skin biopsies, and specimen sample usually present no problems.

—Most Native Americans have some prohibitions about handling the dead, and therefore would not likely consent to an autopsy.

—Family planning (birth control, rhythm, etc.) is considered an individual choice. However, these methods are not frequently used.

—The acceptance of carrier testing is not known. To date, there have been no compelling reasons for its use on a large sector of the population.

—There is a high incidence of fetal alcohol syndrome and fetal alcohol effects, as well as problems associated with exposure to solvents among Native Americans.

—Although the Native Alaskan Yupik Eskimos have a high incidence of congenital adrenal hyperplasia, there is also increased incidence among the Southwestern tribes.

—In greeting families, it is appropriate to address the maternal grandmother first.

—Be aware of the amount of eye contact that is comfortable for the person and adjust the contact accordingly.

—Navajos and others may not answer questions immediately. Do not interrupt the silence, or interpret it as a loss of attention.

—In disclosing "bad news" to the family, consider relating it as a story. For example, "Another couple we knew were in a similar situation and this occurred. This is no reflection on your family or ancestors."

—Physical comfort or touching will probably not be appropriate.

—Grief is handled quietly, or with the family, not in front of strangers.

—Psychological stress is best handled by recommending a healing ceremony rather than a psychologist or psychiatrist.

—Resources for the family come from internal sources.

—In discussions of genetic problems, visual aids may be used. If an individual objects, inquire as to the reason, so as to develop an appropriate ceremony for curing.

—In taking family histories, do not ask whether a couple is related. Instead, ask to which clan each person belongs. Individuals may refer to each other as sister or brother when they are related not by blood but in a ceremonial way.

REFERENCES

Aberle, D. 1951. The psychosocial analysis of a Hopi life history. *Comparative Psychology Monographs* 21:27–41.

―――. 1966. *The Peyote Religion among the Navajo*. Chicago: Aldine.

Basehart, H. W. 1970. Mescalero Apache band organization and leadership. *Southwest Journal of Anthropology* 26:87–106.

Brown, D. 1970. *Bury My Heart at Wounded Knee*. New York: Holt, Rinehart, and Winston.

Dozier, E. P. 1970. *The Pueblo Indians of North America*. New York: Holt, Rinehart, and Winston.

―――. 1972. The Pueblos of the Southwestern United States. *Journal of the Royal Anthropological Institute* 90:146–60.

Driver, H. E. 1969. *Indians of North America*. Chicago: University of Chicago Press.

Dutton, B. P. 1975. *Indians of the American Southwest*. Englewood Cliffs, N.J.: Prentice Hall.

Folsom, F. 1973. *Red Power on the Rio Grande: The Native American Revolution of 1680*. Chicago: Follett.

Forbes, J. P. 1960. *Apache, Navaho, and Spaniard*. Norman: University of Oklahoma Press.

Gifford, E. W. 1940. Cultural element distributions: XII. *Apache Pueblo Anthropological Records* 4:110–16 .

Goodwin, G. 1942. *The Social Organization of the Western Apache*. Tucson: University of Arizona Press.

Haile, B. 1938. Navajo chantways and ceremonials. *American Anthropologist* 40:639–52.

Haley, J. L. 1981. *Apaches: A History and Culture Portrait*. Garden City, N.Y.: Doubleday.

Hammerschlag, C. A. 1988. *The Dancing Healers*. New York: Harper & Row.

Hester, J. 1962. Early Navajo migrations and acculturation in the Southwest. *Papers in Anthropology* 6:47–63.

Hultkrantz, A. 1979. *Religions of the American Indians*. Berkeley: University of California Press.

Kennard, E. A. 1937. Hopi reactions to death. *American Anthropologist* 39:97–104.

Kluckhohn, C. 1962. *Navajo Witchcraft*. Boston: Beacon Press.

Kluckhohn, C., and Leighton, D. 1962. *The Navaho*. Rev. ed. Garden City, N.Y.: Natural History Library.

Leighton, D. 1966. *People of the Middle Place: A Study of the Zuni Indians*. New Haven: Human Relations Area Files.

Levy, J. E. 1974. *Navajo Health Concepts and Behaviors: The Role of the Anglo Medical Man in the Navajo Healing Process*. A report to the U.S. Public Health Service, Indian Health Systems, Bethesda, Md.

Levy, J. E., Neutra, R., and Parker, D. 1987. *Hand Trembling, Frenzy Witchcraft, and Moth Madness: A Study of Navajo Seizure Disorders*. Tucson: University of Arizona Press.

Locke, R. F. 1989. *The Book of the Navajo,* 4th ed. Los Angeles: Mankind Publishing.

Locust, C. 1985a. *Apache Beliefs about Unwellness and Handicaps.* Monograph, Native American Research and Training Center. Tucson: University of Arizona.

———. 1985b. *Hopi Beliefs about Unwellness and Handicaps.* Monograph, Native American Research and Training Center. Tucson: University of Arizona.

———. 1986. *Yoqui Beliefs about Unwellness and Handicaps.* Monograph, Native American Research and Training Center. Tucson: University of Arizona.

Melody, M. 1977. *Apaches: A Critical Bibliography.* New York: Chelsea House.

Morgan, W. 1982. *Coyote Tales.* Bureau of Indian Affairs, Navajo Life Series. Washington, D.C.: GPO.

Navajo Tribal Council and Save the Children Federation. 1987. *Technical Report: A Path to Peace of Mind: Providing Exemplary Services to Navajo Children with Developmental Disabilities and Their Families.* Window Rock, Ariz.: Navajo Tribal Council and Save the Children Federation.

Opler, M. E. 1965. *An Apache Life-way.* New York: Cooper Square.

Parsons, E. C. 1916. A few Zuni death beliefs and practices. *American Anthropologist* 18:245–96.

———. 1917. All Souls Day at Zuni, Acoma, and Laguna. *Journal of American Folklore* 30:495–96.

Paul, N., and Kavanagh, L. 1990. National symposium on genetic services for underserved populations. *Birth Defects* 26:1–290.

Schmitt, M., and Brown, D. 1968. *Fighting Indians of the West.* New York: Bonanza Books.

Strong, W. D. 1927. An analysis of Southwestern society. *American Anthropologist* 29:1–61.

Talayesva, D. C. 1942. *Sun Chief: The Autobiography of a Hopi Indian.* New Haven: Yale University Press.

Thompson, L., and Joseph, A. 1944. *The Hopi Way.* New York: Russell and Russell.

Titiev, M. 1971. *Old Oraibi: A Study of the Hopi Indians of Third Mesa.* Harvard University, Peabody Museum of American Archaeology and Ethnology Papers, vol. 22, no. 1. Cambridge: Harvard University Press.

Underhill, R. M. 1948. Ceremonial patterns in the greater Southwest. *Memories of the American Ethnological Society* 13:67–68.

———. 1965. *Red Man's Religion.* Chicago: University of Chicago Press.

U.S. Bureau of the Census, Economics and Statistics Administration. 1993. *We, the First Americans.* Washington, D.C.: GPO.

U.S. Department of Health and Human Services, Centers for Disease Control. 1989. Leading major congenital malformations among minority groups in the United States, 1981–1986. *Journal of the American Medical Association* 261:205–9.

U.S. Department of Health and Human Services, Indian Health Service. 1990. *Trends in Indian Health.* Washington, D.C.: GPO.

Versluis, A. 1993. *Native American Traditions.* Rockport, Mass.: Element.

Waters, F. 1977. *Book of the Hopi.* New York: Viking Press.

5

Traditional Chinese Culture

Jack H. Jung, M.D.

Until this century, China represented a nation with four to five thousand years of history and relative cultural stability. Only in this century has significant migration to North America occurred. Chinese people presently in North America vary in geographic origin, spoken language, and economic means. However, they often share common aspects of Chinese culture, which can influence their perception of Western medicine and genetic counseling. This chapter will briefly review the recent history, migration patterns, and culture-specific attitudes of the Chinese in relationship to the clinical practice of medical genetics in North America today.

HISTORY

Mainland China is a geographically vast country that covers an area of 9.6 million square kilometers. The country is divided into twenty-two provinces and administered as five autonomous regions. Recent estimates of the population are at more than 1 billion (representing one of every four people in the world).

North American families of Chinese ancestry may be diverse in geographic origin and vary considerably in their time of initial emigration. This composition, over time, has been influenced by many events in recent history. Significant Chinese immigration to North America began in the middle 1800s. The majority of early immigrants came from the province of Guangdong, in southern China. Within Guangdong province, the immigrants specifically came from the agriculturally based Sze Yap (Four Counties) region. Although this area is subtropical in climate and usually experiences long growing seasons, it provided only basic levels of subsistence for its population base.

Although many circumstances encouraged these Chinese people to seek opportunities in the New World, a major factor was the failure of agricultural production in the Sze Yap region to keep pace with the rapidly increasing population. The first Opium War (1839–42) and the Taiping Rebellion (1854–68) also disrupted agricultural production. The unsettling result of all these events was that many male peasants were forced to leave their rural environment for urban centers such as Guangzhou (previously called Canton), the capital of Guangdong province.

During this time, there was increasing contact between China and the West, with Guangzhou figuring prominently in this interface. Guangzhou is situated at the mouth of the Pearl River and became established as a major port. In 1757, Guangzhou was recognized as the sole Chinese port to trade with the West (Yee, 1989). The timely influx of peasants from nearby Sze Yap, many of whom were surviving under desperate conditions, made them prime candidates for the work force being actively recruited by Westerners for projects in North America. Stories related to the vast resources and potential opportunities of North America fostered their dreams and ambitions for success. The name given to North America by the Chinese translates literally as "Gold Mountain," reflecting this perception of wealth. Accounts of their early, and often arduous, involvement with the construction of the railroads and gold mining are well chronicled (Morton, 1980; Con et al., 1982; Yee, 1989). Many of these Chinese laborers even-tually sought to establish families in North America, but restrictive immigration policies seriously challenged these efforts. However, there are presently some Chinese descendants in North America who represent the third or fourth generation of the early settlers from the mid-1800s.

The events of World War II influenced another significant period of immigration. In China, the conflict intensified the long history of warring with Japan. Full-scale Sino-Japanese war broke out in 1937 and did not subside until the resolution of World War II. During this war the Chinese found themselves allied with the United States and Canada. This, in turn, led to the relaxation of citizenship and immigration policies in the postwar period. Individuals who became naturalized citizens were allowed to apply for immigration privileges for family members who remained in China.

In China, internal conflicts also influenced patterns of migration. Chiang Kai-shek led the Nationalists against Mao Zedong and the Communists in a civil war that ended with a Communist victory in 1949. Events associated with the Communist takeover contributed to the flight of some families to Hong Kong for refuge. Most of these families were from nearby Guangdong. Those lucky enough to have ties with North America were more likely to be candidates for immigration. Many of these were families from the Sze Yap region whose relatives had earlier tried to establish themselves in North America. In the period immediately after World War II and into the 1950s, immigrants from the Sze Yap region continued to constitute the majority of Chinese in major metropolitan centers such as San Francisco and Vancouver. Their spoken language reflected the Four Counties' distinct dialects: Toi San, Sun Wui, Hoi Ping, and Yin Ping (in decreasing order of frequency).

Beginning in the 1960s and continuing to the present, individuals of Cantonese origin, primarily from Hong Kong, have represented the largest number of Chinese immigrants to North America. North America remains an attractive destination, with its high quality educational institutions, generally high standards of living, and democratic society. This last factor is not insignificant, given the uncertainties that presently exist with the impending takeover of Hong Kong by China in 1997. These Cantonese-speaking individuals presently comprise the majority of North Americans of Chinese descent. However, the fabric of the community is still changing.

Recent political changes in mainland China have allowed for another wave of immigrants. Many have come to North America for various Chinese government-sponsored academic pursuits. Mandarin is the official language in China today and is the dialect most commonly spoken by this group of visitors or immigrants. Given their educational background, they often have adequate communication skills in the English language. This group is beginning to make a significant impact on Chinese communities in America. However, at present, Cantonese is still the dialect most commonly encountered in North America. There exist sufficient differences in spoken language to make oral communication difficult or impossible between some dialects. However, Chinese people share a common written language.

From this brief summary of immigration patterns, one can appreciate that the individuals of Chinese origin presently in North America are not homogeneous in dialect, language, or socioeconomic levels. However, they share a number of cultural similarities, many of which are still prominent in their value systems in North America today. Predictably, these characteristics are generally more evident in newer immigrants.

RELIGION

The two major religions of China are Buddhism and Taoism. A minority follow Muslim and Christian religions (primarily Roman Catholic). The Buddhist and Taoist religions particularly stress concepts related to the importance of the family and striving for a long and happy life through elimination of desires and aggressive tendencies. After the Communist takeover in 1949 and particularly during the Cultural Revolution in the middle 1960s, religious practice was actively discouraged. More recently, religious observances have become more tolerated.

The values of Confucianism and ancestor worship also inform social values, which include respect for superiors and elders, benevolence, filial piety, and loyalty, and have helped to maintain social and domestic order. These beliefs are especially prevalent among older Chinese. These individuals or couples are often more comfortable with accepting directive suggestions for health care management. However, strong beliefs in more traditional methods of medical practice may counterbalance such values. A sensitivity to and appreciation of the religious background of a family will become increasingly important in determining genetic mangement options, especially as more Chinese adopt Christian religions.

FAMILY

Confucian philosophy emphasizes the importance of the family in establishing societal harmony. Family stability is attained through a patriarchal structure, generally with the greatest respect and authority given to the eldest male member. Age, sex, and generational status determine roles. Elders are respected. The head of the house is the father, and females are subservient to males. Historically, families became organized in networks, or clans, based on common ancestors with the same surname. These clans offered greater organization, resources, and support systems for individuals or their families, giving all members a sense of belonging to a larger societal unit. Today, the welfare of the family is still placed above individual needs and desires. Public admission of problems is not the norm, since this would bring shame and cause the family to "lose face." Therefore, illegitimacy, abortion, and divorce are rare in the traditional family. Nonpaternity is highly unusual. Although the government of the People's Republic of China strongly encourages small families (through financial incentives and coercion), the tendency to have larger families is seen in other countries.

With many families having relied on agriculture for subsistence or their livelihoods, male children became regarded, in many families, as more important than females. The failure of a couple to have a male child also meant that a family's lineage, by surname, would come to an end. This is still a common concern among couples who do not accept the values of equality between the sexes. Grandparents' expectations and pressures also need to be considered, as they are more likely to have antiquated values.

Mothers of Chinese ancestry are said to have high expectations for themselves and their children. This would certainly place greater burden on them if a child were not healthy or had a significant disability. The responsibility for a healthy pregnancy and child was also the woman's, so in cases where the pregnancy outcomes were less than ideal, the mother would receive more than her share of suspicion and potential blame.

Child-rearing among traditional Chinese families is almost the sole responsibility of the mother. Children may also receive a great deal of attention, as it is regarded as extremely important to nurture them and encourage development to their potential. If health problems exist, the family will predictably vigorously pursue possible treatments.

It is becoming less common for three generations of a family to live under one roof. Traditionally, the eldest son was responsible for taking care of his parents in their old age, and the family was expected to provide for any sick individuals. However, families of Chinese origin are willing to recognize and accept any social programs or external support systems perceived to be of potential benefit.

Family names are important in Chinese culture, as evidenced by the desire of many couples to have a male child. A person's name is structured as three characters, with the family name first, followed by given names. The given names usually signify important traits that the parents wish their child to have. In interviews, it is proper to address adults by Mr. or Mrs., as opposed to their given name. Given names are usually reserved for intrafamilial use or among the closest friends.

COMMUNICATION

Chinese philosophy emphasizes the importance of harmonious interpersonal relationships. The success of a physician or genetic counselor engaged in genetic discussions with a family will depend on numerous factors, which may be culture-specific tendencies.

Traditionally, Chinese people are reluctant to talk about personal feelings, especially to people outside of the family. This emphasis on privacy may make it difficult to ascertain whether social problems exist. Another topic that may be discomforting is the open discussion of sexual matters, unless it is seen as relevant and important to the presenting problem. These tendencies could increase the challenge of determining accurate histories related to infertility, miscarriage, or sexual dysfunction.

Older-generation Chinese people may tend not to display emotions openly in the presence of strangers, making it difficult to appreciate whether the consultand is fully aware or accepting of the information given in genetic counseling situations.

The Chinese are not known to be openly physically demonstrative with unfamiliar individuals. In counseling situations, a counselor should be aware that physical contact (such as an arm around a shoulder or holding a hand), as a demonstration of empathy and support, may not be comfortably accepted or appreciated.

BELIEFS ABOUT HEALTH

Most families realize the importance of hereditary factors in determining health and disease. It is not uncommon for a family history of severe disorders to be an important consideration in the choice of a spouse. There may also be a tendency to assume that a familial problem is genetic until proven otherwise.

In mainland China today, there exists official recognition of traditional Chinese and Western-oriented modalities of health care in both education and practice. It is not surprising that, in many large North American cities,

Chinese herbalists or acupuncture specialists find an eager clientele. It is not that Western medicine is looked down on, but that more traditional methods of treatment are perceived to have potential for benefit. The comfort of communicating with a physician in a native tongue also cannot be overlooked as a factor in the choice of a traditional approach to health problems and their treatment. It is common to prefer a combination of traditional Chinese and Western medical practices.

The belief in the yin-yang theory of a natural balance underlies the traditional Chinese concept of maintaining health. (This subject cannot be adequately addressed in this chapter.) Within these concepts of health maintenance and disease causation is the tendency to believe in an organic cause of any medical problem.

IMPLICATIONS FOR GENETIC SERVICES

Some traditional Chinese beliefs may influence the utilization of genetic services. *Feng shui,* which literally means "wind and water," is the art of location, orientation, and design of physical structures to aid achieving proper harmony and balance. Positive feng shui is thought to ward off evil spirits and promote good health and prosperity. For example, triangular shapes are considered bad luck and are therefore not used in house construction. Doors should not open directly facing traffic; it is believed that this would allow evil spirits direct access to the building. Additionally, the best position for a building is facing water, with the rear of the building to the mountains, to encourage prosperity and offer protection to those living within the structure.

Other folk beliefs and superstitions involve numbers and colors. The number four is considered bad luck, as it sounds like the word for "dead." The number eight is highly regarded, as it sounds like the word for "good luck." One who was born on 8–8–88 would be considered extremely lucky, a blessed one destined for a prosperous life. Red is a "good" color, whereas white is the color of mourning. Imagine the implications for a new immigrant or older-generation Chinese person if she or he attended a modern triangular-shaped clinic building, located at 444 Fourth Avenue, and all the personnel working in this clinic wore white coats. Given a choice, Chinese immigrants would not use this facility.

Any difficulties with oral communication will quickly become apparent. In selecting an interpreter, it may not be satisfactory merely to request a person capable of speaking Chinese. At the least, a distinction should be made between the two major dialects of Chinese: Cantonese (and some similar dialects) and Mandarin. Some individuals have a good command of both dialects. When an interpreter is required, it is probably better to choose one who is the same sex and age as (or older than) the consultand. Better success may relate to the respect accorded to an older individual, who may be perceived to have greater experience. In nonemergency situations, where there is time to plan, it is probably best to leave the choice of an interpreter to the patient or family, if at all possible. Most recent genetic terminology, short of those terms specific to recombinant DNA technology, have a Chinese translation.

The geneticist or genetic counselor should be aware of possible sensitivities of some Chinese people to certain ethnic groups. Strained ethnic relationships during times of war are not easily forgotten by people directly or indirectly involved. For example, Chinese people who lived through the most recent Japanese incursion into China may have difficulty trusting or dealing with a Japanese person. There may also exist some animosity or distrust between individuals of different political orientations (e.g., Nationalist versus Communist).

News regarding severe birth defects or mental retardation will usually be viewed as catastrophic. Many new immigrants and older individuals will feel a sense of shame or inferiority in these circumstances and the tendency will be for less openness when dealing with people outside of the family. It is very important that clients be made aware that matters will be handled in a confidential manner, as it will determine the success of continued interactions.

In any genetic counseling situation there exists the potential for blame. If a genetic trait or disease is determined to be of maternal origin, the counselor needs to be aware of the risk for excessive blame to be placed on the mother or her family. Even when there is no maternal factor (such as the genetic determinant of a child's sex), the mother may be deemed to have failed. Where a paternal contribution to a genetic disorder is recognized, it should not come as a surprise if the male does not accept this unless there is convincing objective evidence. In situations where there is no easy explanation of disease etiology, there may be a tendency to blame certain life events, persons, or bad spirits.

Although marital pressures and disharmony may be intensified during health-related crises, separation or divorce is not a likely outcome, as it is not socially acceptable in Chinese culture. This is not meant to imply that a genetic counselor should not consider the possible benefits of a social worker in particularly stressful situations. The traditional family plays a strong role in coping with serious illness. The decision to seek help from outside the family will depend on the availability of services and the family's socioeconomic status.

The issue of nondirective counseling may be a problem for recent immigrants of limited education or from strongly socialistic systems, such as exist in mainland China. Their life style might have previously been one of following orders and instructions given by individuals in positions of authority, such as physicians, so the opportunity to be involved in decision-making processes may represent a new challenge.

Possibly because of the Chinese tendency to believe in an organic cause of any medical problem, there may also be the expectation for potential treatment. Oral communication or counseling alone may not be perceived as effective unless it is backed up by practical management options. The level of understanding or acceptance of counseling or management options will be determined in part by the educational background of the patient or family.

No studies have shown any cross-cultural differences in the acceptance of newer reproductive technologies. It is likely that these technologies would be acceptable to Chinese couples, especially if addressing a problem of infertility. In fact increasing capabilities to determine fetal sex might prompt unwarranted requests for technologies involving fetal sexing or fetal preselection.

Acquiring Genetic Information

If a search of medical records is undertaken to verify a diagnosis or acquire other information, the counselor needs to be aware of possible inaccuracies of name or date of birth. Families of Chinese origin have not been prone to keeping detailed records of ancestors or family history. A health care professional may encounter problems in acquiring information regarding correct name and age from individuals who emigrated to North America many years ago. The Chinese custom of referring to an individual with the family name preceding the given names was mentioned earlier. Immigration papers would often document the name in an incorrect fashion, increasing the risk of confusing which name was the surname. There was also variability in the transliteration of Chinese surnames into English. For example, the surnames Wong and Huang represent the same Chinese family name but became different English names because of the Chinese dialectal differences in pronunciation. Language problems at the time of immigration may also contribute to inaccuracy in the recording of names. Incorrect birth date information may also arise because of differences in calendars. Many new immigrants and older Chinese still rely on the lunar calendar. Inaccuracies may be purely unintentional, although there are past examples of false documentation of name or date of birth to satisfy immigration policies in certain jurisdictions.

It is worthwhile for health care professionals to know, while obtaining pedigree information, that the Chinese definition of consanguineous relationships is consistent with the genetic definition. Consanguineous marriages (and even marriages between couples with the same family name) are actively discouraged, although why this custom evolved is not well documented in Chinese folklore. In remote rural parts of China, first-cousin marriages may be grudgingly accepted due to the practical limitations of a lack of available partners, but this would be uncommon.

Genetic Diseases

The thalassemias are the most common genetic problem in the Chinese population. The estimated incidence of α thalassemia 1 and 2 in the Chinese is between 5 and 10 percent (Kendall, 1982). Hemoglobin H disease and hemoglobin Bart's hydrops fetalis are also well recognized. Approximately 1 percent of Chinese are thought to have β thalassemia minor (Huntsman, 1982; Weatherall et al., 1989).

The list of less prominent genetic conditions includes alcoholism and fetal alcohol syndrome. In the long history of China, it is quite remarkable that alcoholism has never been a notable social or medical problem. Studies have demonstrated biological differences in the enzymes responsible for the metabolism of alcohol. These genetic polymorphisms prevalent in the Asian population do not predispose to high rates of consumption of alcohol. It is not understood how the social control mechanism of traditional Chinese society may have influenced these behaviors. With increasing Westernization of families of Chinese descent, it would not be surprising to see the rate of alcohol-related pathologies increase. With the rate of alcoholism so low, it is predictable that the incidence of fetal alcohol syndrome is also low. It has not been demonstrated whether any other enzyme polymorphisms would either increase or decrease teratogenic potential.

The major psychoses are less prevalent in the Chinese population than in other cultures (Lin, 1983). This may represent underdiagnosis, due either to differences in the medical or psychiatric diagnostic criteria or to a reflection of the cultural tendency to keep personal matters and feelings to oneself or immediate family members.

CONCLUSION

The immigration of Chinese people to North America is ongoing. They represent a heterogeneous group whose members differ in dialect, level of education, socioeconomic means, and degree of Westernization. In dealing with any ethnic group, health care providers should be sensitive to culture-specific attitudes and needs, particularly for those individuals or families requiring genetic services. In the case of traditional Chinese, providers should remember that the eldest male has authority. In all interactions, nonverbal communication and formality are very important. Recognition of these and other culture-specific issues should help increase the chances for successful patient management.

SUMMARY

—Greet individuals as Mr. or Mrs. Remember, the family name is written first. Greet elders first.

—Spend a few moments establishing rapport by making "small talk."

—Avoid physical touching for comforting.

—Explain what will happen in the counseling session before beginning. Emphasize, up front, that no medication will be given.

—Allow the family to make decisions in a group, consulting other family members if necessary. In traditional families, the eldest male has the most authority.

—Inquire about the patient's age—specifically, how the age was calculated. Remember, there may be differences in age calculation as well as errors upon immigration.

—Choose an interpreter who speaks the correct Chinese dialect—usually Mandarin or Cantonese. Discuss the choice of an interpreter with the family, if possible. Avoid using children as interpreters, unless the family requests this.

—Adoptions are rare.

—Autopsy is generally seen as both irrelevant and expensive.

—Artificial insemination by donor is probably not acceptable to most. However, GIFT and in vitro fertilization may be employed to help with fertility problems.

—Carrier testing and other technologies may create a potential for blame, especially on the mother. Emphasize the importance of "no fault."

—Avoid wearing a white coat to the session.

—Do not schedule a clinic on Chinese New Year (late January to early February). Be aware that many American calendars will not note the Chinese New Year.

—There are no general prohibitions against photos, and the use of visual aids is appropriate and helpful.

—Many generations of people of Chinese origin in North America are acculturated. Determine each patient's own degree of assimilation into Western culture.

—Nonverbal body language is important. Caring, polite gestures can be "read."

—Family histories may be incomplete and mental illness is not well recognized or acknowledged.

REFERENCES

Con, H., Con, R. J., Johnson, G., Wickberg, E., and Willmott, W. E. 1982. *From China to Canada: A History of the Chinese Communities in Canada.* Wickberg, E. (ed.) Toronto: McClelland and Stewart.

Decary, F. 1982. Neonatal alloimmune thrombocytopenia. *Medicine North America* 26: 2553–56.

Fisher, N. S. 1992. Ethnocultural approaches to genetics. *Pediatric Clinics of North America* 39:55–64.

Huntsman, R. G. 1982. Hemoglobinopathies. *Medicine North America* 26:2529–35.

Kendall, A. G. 1982. Thalassemias. *Medicine North America* 26:2536–45.

Lin, T. Y. 1983. Psychiatry and Chinese culture. *Western Journal of Medicine* 139:862–67.

Marston, D. 1992. Challenge of cross-cultural medicine. *Physicians Management Manuals* 16:18–25.

Morton, J. 1980. *In the Sea of Sterile Mountains: The Chinese in British Columbia.* Vancouver: J. J. Douglas.

Weatherall, D. J., Clegg, J. B., Higgs, D. R., and Wood, W. G. 1989. The hemoglobinopathies. In Scriver, C. R., Beaudet, A. L., Sly, W. S., and Valle, D. (eds.), *The Metabolic Basis of Inherited Disease,* 6th ed., p. 2332. Toronto: McGraw-Hill Information Services.

Worsley, P. 1982. Non-Western medical systems. *Annual Review of Anthropology* 11:315–48.

Yee, P. 1989. *Saltwater City: An Illustrated History of the Chinese in Vancouver.* Vancouver: Douglas and McIntyre.

6

Traditional Japanese Culture

Marie D. Strazar, Ph.D.,
and Nancy L. Fisher, R.N., M.D., M.P.H.

Japan is an archipelago in the Pacific Ocean that extends almost 1,774 miles from north to south. The islands are separated from the Asian continent by the Sea of Japan. The four main islands are Hokkaido, Honshu, Shikoku, and Kyushu. Narrow fissures and valleys characterize Japanese mountain chains. The climate is mainly temperate; however, the southwestern area of the country is often hit by typhoons.

The Japanese population is estimated at 121 million, with the majority of the people concentrated along the Pacific seaboard, specifically in the Kanto and Kansai plains, the locations of Tokyo and Osaka, respectively. The dominant ethnic group is Japanese, though Koreans make up 1 percent of the population and there are small groups of Ainu (Japanese of Caucasian background) scattered in the northern parts of the country, predominantly in Hokkaido. The major language is Japanese and the illiteracy rate is 1 percent or less.

HISTORY AND MIGRATION

Scholars continue to debate the origin of the Japanese people, be it in Southeast Asia or in the larger Asian land mass to the west. The presence of the Ainu further complicates the debate. Early history is dominated by a clan period, with emperors and empresses as absolute rulers. The Taika reforms brought a system of village and governmental organization that depended on loyalty to local officials. There was no capital at that time and the court moved from town to town. In 710 a permanent court was established at Nara. During the Heian period, beginning in 784, the capital was established at Kyoto. This was a time of strife, as the government tried to gain control over local officials. Concomitant with the rise of military power came feudalism. This era of constant upheaval and fighting ended in the sixteenth century when unification was achieved. Oda Nobunaga, Toyotomi Hideyoshi, and Tokugawa Ieyasu were men of exceptional abilities, both military and political. Their shogunates provided a stable base for the country, despite civil disruptions and minor foreign influences (Japan was officially closed to foreigners as of 1603).

After 1853, when Japan was officially "opened" once again to foreigners, foreign influence exacerbated domestic problems that led to the downfall of the feudal system as well as the shogunate. The Meiji period, beginning in 1868, brought not only the restoration of the emperor to full power but also a constitutional movement and industrialization. The growth of basic manufacturing was promoted, along with many other changes in education, agriculture, and the military. The population also continued to grow and food shortages became more common.

In the 1860s, and more extensively in the 1880s, Japanese people began to immigrate to Canada, the United States (including Hawaii), and South America. They often experienced discrimination, harassment, and punishment. As more and more Asians came, an anti-Oriental atmosphere developed in North America, giving rise to the phrase "the yellow peril." In Canada, an anti-Asian riot in 1907 led to legislation restricting immigration to Canada and the control of emigration by the Japanese government. At the same time there was a "gentleman's agreement" to decrease the number of immigrants into the United States. In 1913 California passed the Alien Land Law, forbidding foreign nationals to own land. Propaganda and feelings against the Japanese had become so intense that the Asian Land Law was passed to prevent the Japanese from controlling farmland. In reality, there were 11 million acres of agricultural land in California and Japanese people owned a little more than 12 thousand acres.

In Japan, some believed the rise of the military could solve economic problems. Immigration to many nations was slowed or stopped, contributing to domestic hardship. Military proponents eventually rose in power and the government made concessions to them, thereby eliciting foreign distrust. Aggressive acts by the Japanese military in Manchuria in the 1930s did not help foreign relations. The U.S. response to Japanese interest in Indochina was to impose an oil embargo. Negotiations between the two countries commenced, but the Japanese military had its own solution. This predicament served as the catalyst for the attack on Pearl Harbor.

The attack on Pearl Harbor increased suspicion about people of Japanese ancestry living in the United States and Canada, especially those on the West Coast, and many were rounded up, relocated, and confined in camps in noncoastal areas. For years after World War II, Americans of Japanese origin experienced discrimination and were underemployed, given their educational status. Immigration into Canada and the United States virtually stopped between 1920 and 1960 because of laws limiting Asian immigration. However, the 1980 U.S. Census revealed a population of Americans of Japanese ancestry of more than seven hundred thousand individuals. By the 1990s this population had increased to more than eight hundred thousand.

Each generation of Japanese immigrants to the United States or elsewhere has a specific designation. This is comparable to the usual generational designation for anyone who migrated or whose ancestors migrated (for example, it is common to say that someone is a third-generation or fifth-generation American).

First-generation Japanese immigrants are called *issei* (in Japanese, literally, "first generation"). Although many emigrated to escape conditions in Japan, to seek work, and to improve their standard of living, they maintained many of their Japanese traditions and at the same time adapted to American ways. As with most immigrants anywhere in the world, they tended to form their own communities. They were subjected to considerable discrimination and racism, and to the consequent psychological stress. They were perceived as resisting acculturation. However, their strong hold to many of their own traditions could have been more a reaction to the hostile treatment they received than to personal obstinacy.

The *nisei* are the second generation. They were born in North America or in the country to which their parents migrated. These individuals grew up in the society of their birthplace but were taught traditional Japanese values and beliefs at home. They spoke Japanese, since it was their parents' language, but were bilingual, since they also grew up speaking the language of their birthplace. Again, typical of the second generation of any immigrant group, they felt an urgency to acculturate in order to demonstrate their "Americanness" and be accepted among their peers.

Kibei or *kika nisei* were born in the United States or another country and sent to Japan between the ages of eight and fourteen, usually for education. Most then returned to their birthplace. Kibei often found themselves not fully accepted in either country or culture; however, many returned and adjusted quite easily to life in North America. Many of them proved invaluable as instructors in the U.S. military during World War II.

The third generation, *sansei,* were reared by nisei and are as acculturated to Western culture as any third-generation group. Many retain their ethnic identity and are interested in their family backgrounds and histories, though few know or speak Japanese.

Yonsei and *gosei,* the fourth and fifth generations, are "totally" acculturated, as is typical for any ethnic group. This fact contradicts the prejudice that leads other Americans to assume that assimilation is not possible for Japanese, given that their native culture is so very different from Western culture. However, in keeping with the high value that Japanese people place on success and education, acculturation was and is both natural and inevitable.

Since the 1960s, new immigrants have come to North America. These individuals have left the country of their birth to explore entrepreneurial opportunities, to free themselves from the restrictions of the Japanese social system, or to pursue higher education, since access to Japanese universities is extremely competitive.

Today, there are also many temporary residents from Japan living in the United States and Canada. These are usually employees of Japanese companies who are sent on business or students at American colleges and universities.

RELIGION

Shintoism and Buddhism, to which more than 80 percent of the population adhere, are the major religions of Japan. Christianity is also well established in Japan, and many Americans of Japanese descent are Christian. However, funerals are likely to be Buddhist ceremonies, especially for issei and nisei. Birth and marriage are often colored by Shinto rituals, though this is less so for yonsei and gosei. Like the church in Western culture, the temple (Buddhist) or shrine (Shinto) is also part of social organization.

In Shintoism the blessings of the gods are obtained for good fortune in future events and there are ceremonies to bless infants, children, and weddings. Talismans are used for a variety of reasons, including health-related functions. Buddhism, in contrast, is much more philosophical and is not based on a belief in a particular god. Buddhists are encouraged to achieve an ultimate state of enlightenment. There are Buddhist ceremonies to honor ancestors and a family altar may occupy a place of honor in the home. Additionally today, many young women go to the Buddhist temple to visit *mizuko jizo* (small figures representing the unborn) because of fear of cursing present or future family life. The original concept is associated with stillborns and miscarriages, but now includes abortuses as well. These "unborn" were stranded on the banks of the river that separated the worlds of life and death. Too young to have souls, they needed guidance across to the land of the dead.

Buddhists believe in reincarnation and have ceremonies at the time of death which provide comfort and reconciliation. A wake is held the evening before cremation. On the seventh and forty-ninth days after a death, services are held to bid happiness for the dead. In general, individuals prefer to die at home. Grief is private, so public expression of grief is not common. Personal bereavement may be expressed by a small smile and announcement of the death.

All Japanese religions honor the family. Special holidays celebrate children, adulthood (age fifteen), and aged persons. In summer, the holiday of *o-bon* is a time to return to one's hometown to visit the graves of ancestors. Given the homage paid to ancestors in these traditional religions, it is natural for Japanese people to place a high value on heritage, filial piety, and the moral obligation to others over self. In Japanese society, individual concerns are secondary to concerns for the group.

FAMILY

The traditional Japanese family structure is patriarchal and it is the husband's role to work and provide for the family. If he is the eldest male in his family, he is also responsible for his aging parents. The wife's duty is to serve her husband and to raise the children. All care of the children is the wife's responsibility. She also must care for those who are ill in the family (often including the extended family) and manage the household. It has been traditional for women in Japan to be passive and submissive. It was the mother-in-law's job to see that her daughter-in-law carried out her duties.

Amae is a term that describes the mother-child relationship, as well as other relationships, consisting of affection, the encouragement of dependency, and rendering emotional satisfaction. Japanese parents are quite permissive with children until they reach six or seven years of age, when strict discipline begins with schooling. Sleeping arrangements are often more crowded and intimate than is typical in Western cultures, due in part to the small size of living quarters in Japan. It is not unusual in this situation for young children of both sexes to share the same room. At one time, age calculation was also different than Western calculation: a child was considered to be one year old at birth.

Allegiance to family is all important. Some postulate that this developed in feudal times as a means to ensure familial safety. In modern times the racism Japanese people experienced in countries to which they immigrated may have served to reinforce this traditional value. Family members are encouraged to keep family concerns at home and not divulge problems to outsiders. It has also been important for members of the family not to shame the family.

Matchmakers *(nakoodo)* have often been used to make a match of individuals according to socioeconomic status and compatibility. A matchmaker's responsibility is taken very seriously; it is not casual. The purpose of marriage is considered to be procreation and it is common to believe that the development of love takes time. The divorce rate in Japan is low. It has been common for husbands in Japan to have mistresses. This practice has had a significant impact on the family financially, since the mistress often has a separate home that must be maintained. In the past, if a husband fathered a child by his mistress, the mistress could be brought to the man's house, but she was commonly treated as a servant.

Abortion is not condoned, but it is not uncommon for a couple of reasons. First, an unwed mother brings great shame to the family. Second, there is a great emphasis on population control in modern Japan. Adoption has become more common in recent times, though traditionally if a family did not have a son, they would often adopt a boy to carry on the family name.

Education is very prized in modern Japan. Education is highly competitive, since positions with companies often depend on which university one has attended. Graduates of choice universities get better jobs. Therefore, young children may go to class during the day and receive tutoring or attend additional classes in the evening. In the past, this concern was usually directed toward male children, since women were not expected to have careers outside the home. Girls were taught to suppress their ideas, whereas boys were socialized to be assertive and successful. Today, however, many women train for jobs and work until, or, increasingly, after, marriage.

Jobs have generally been considered to be held for a lifetime. In turn, the employee is expected to be loyal to the company. Because a job means security, it has come to define status, social encounters, and future educational opportunities for one's children. Health care is also a part of this security.

COMMUNICATION

In Japan, formality, including forms of indirect communication, is important in communication. An individual's family name is used in addressing that individual; it is also placed first when written or spoken, unlike the Western practice of indicating it last. Titles are important and are included as a matter of course in introductions. Bowing indicates respect and is used in both greeting and bidding farewell. The higher the status of the recipient, the deeper the bow expected. Avoiding eye contact has also been considered a demonstration of respect. Many modern Japanese, however, are aware of the Western preference for direct eye contact. Still, many Japanese people prefer downcast eyes, shifting the glasses, or doing a "lighthouse" sweep.

In Japan a nod of the head indicates attentiveness, *not* agreement. The words "I understand" also do not necessarily mean agreement. Since the expression of emotion is not encouraged, a smile can mean joy, confusion, concealed rage, or many other things. Silence often occurs in response to embarrassing situations.

CULTURE

Japanese society is organized on the basis of a strong sense of duty. Social obligations and responsibilities are very important, as are *enryo,* reserve and constraint, and conformity. Individuals are expected to follow conventional behavior and maintain a strict allegiance to rules and regulations. Suffering and hard work are generally considered part of character-building. Respect for elders is valued highly and their opinions are sought in many situations, including health care. Since duty is among the highest virtues, one may resort to suicide if one fails or brings other great shame upon the family. In fact, it can even be considered one's duty to commit suicide under such circumstances.

Superstitious beliefs are common, and knowledgeable persons pick lucky days for weddings, house building, and other important events. The numbers four and nine are unlucky: the word for four in Japanese sounds like the word for death, and the word *nine* in Japanese sounds like the word for suffering. There are also ages associated with risks and celebrations occur when one passes each of those ages: for women, they are ages nineteen, thirty-three, and thirty-seven; for men, they are ages twenty-five, forty-two, and sixty-one.

BELIEFS ABOUT HEALTH

The basis for health practices in Japan includes a mixture of traditional medical practice *(kampo)* brought to Japan from China, Shinto beliefs, and Western medicine. Traditional medicine is based on the belief that good health is maintained by attention to diet, exercise, sleep, and good interpersonal relationships. Imbalance in these spectra results in illness.

Polar opposites exist as part of traditional beliefs: *yin* and *yang*. Yin is assigned the following characteristics: female, cold, empty, dark, and negative. Yang is assigned the attributes male, warm, light, and positive. Everything is characterized by both yin and yang, and the two opposites must be kept in balance. Also, one must pay attention to both the environment and one's body, for neither operates in isolation. *Hara,* the stomach, is considered important; there appears to be a great fear about diseases of the stomach. A *haramaki,* a cloth worn around the abdomen, is used for protection by children, elderly persons, and pregnant women. Laborers, such as construction workers, can also be seen wearing a haramaki. The Japanese believe that attention must be paid to diet and appropriate nutrition is said to consist of a proper balance between yin and yang foods. In the past, surgery was not a preferred part of medical treatment since, in accord with the aforementioned beliefs, it upsets the body's normal balance and harmony. Today, however, it is widely accepted.

Traditional health care includes mild medicines, usually made from dried herbs. Mild symptoms are treated early by this means so as not to develop into more severe health problems. Acupuncture is also used as a treatment, as is moxibustion, a heat treatment for stimulation in which small balls of moxa are ignited and placed directly on the skin. These two treatments are used primarily for skeletal and muscular problems. Fever is usually treated by sweating it out with hot drinks and warm blankets. Contrary to Western treatments, which may include a tepid bath, a bath is a leisurely soak, sometimes even a family affair, and is quite different from the Western style of bathing: the actual washing and rinsing are done before the bath. Bathing is usually suspended during illness.

Western medicine brought Japan excellent facilities for health care, mental health care, and health insurance. (Note, however, that prenatal care and delivery are not commonly covered by insurance.) In fact, Western medicine is considered very potent by Japanese standards. Patients seeking medical care for even mild symptoms expect a full examination and treatment. Frequent checkups are common, and a family member may report the patient's status to the physician on a regular basis. Before major health decisions are made, some members in very traditional families may consult with a priest in an attempt to ensure luck.

A physician trained in accord with Western standards has high status and is sought because he or she is expected to know best. Out of deference to the physician, the patient may ask few questions. The Japanese patient tends to agree to almost everything but expects treatment and explanation. Consent forms are not considered necessary. Promptness for appointments is expected.

Japanese women usually prefer a female obstetrician. In Japan, midwives deliver most of the babies, with an obstetrician available if needed. In other health care matters, however, Japanese patients will accept care from a nurse or other health care provider only if the physician has formally authorized it and made that clear to the patients.

Hospital stays often last longer in Japan than in the United States, with family members providing meals, clothing, company, and even some care for the patient. This often means that the health care provider and visitors spend far more time with the patient. Gifts are preferably of a temporal nature, to symbolize that the illness too will abate. A potted plant, for example, would be considered inappropriate because of its association with permanence. The use of gowns with ties and nonsecure closure should be avoided, since they compromise privacy. Since showers are not the preferred method of personal cleansing, the patient may be reluctant to use a shower. (However, showers are increasingly used in Japan, so that reluctance may not surface.)

Talking about sexual matters is embarrassing to both sexes. The male is responsible for contraception. Pregnancy is viewed as a happy time and pregnant women are pampered. It has been the practice traditionally to restrict the intake of spicy and salty foods at about the fifth month of pregnancy. The pregnant woman is expected to be stoic; however, anesthetics are now made available for her use. Circumcision is not performed. The infant's umbilical cord is sprinkled with preservatives after removal and saved in a wooden box.

Children with disabilities are considered a cause for shame and embarrassment, and, therefore, a concern. A couple may be very reluctant to discuss problems related to such a situation. Attention to disabled persons has increased since World War II. Previously, the tendency was to isolate disabled persons in special institutions. Mental illness is also stigmatized and feared in Japan and therefore is not usually discussed openly. Elderly persons may even commit suicide if they perceive themselves to be alienated or "unworthy."

Drinking of alcohol is considered acceptable for men but not for women, though that is changing. So, too, with smoking: many men smoke, but few women have until recently. Nowadays, however, more and more young women are smoking.

IMPLICATIONS FOR GENETIC SERVICES

The family's importance in the Japanese social structure also influences medical practice. Since the individual is responsible for his or her health, seeking a physician can imply individual failure. The physician is considered a skilled technician and a sympathetic assistant in the process of curing, but is not expected to take complete responsibility for a cure. However, the physician is assumed to be the authority figure and the patient will respect the physician and do what is bid. Nonetheless, if there is any family disagreement, this will usually not be indicated. Confrontation of any sort will usually be avoided. The expectation is for treatment.

The patient must perceive that the physician is competent, and formality is extremely important, particularly in interactions with Japanese nationals and recent first-generation immigrants. Titles should be used, particularly at the time of introduction. Patients should be addressed by their last name throughout the period of care, unless they say otherwise. Some will be very anxious to show that they are familiar with the American practice of less formality and use of first names and they will usually comment on that, if that is the case.

A physician should not ask a patient a question that could require a "no" answer; a "what" question is preferable, to avoid any confusion on the physician's part. (Rather than say, "Do you have any questions?" ask "What are your questions?") The patient may be concerned about preserving harmony or not appearing confrontational and may conform his or her answer to achieve that. Even if a Japanese person says "yes," this may not necessarily mean agreement to act. That answer may be only a means of preserving harmony and avoiding upsetting the physician. What is said and what is done are not always the same. Occasionally, the patient may provide misinformation so as not to upset the provider, or may decline to give a straight answer, instead saying something like, "I'll try my best." In addition, the Japanese and English languages differ in how "yes" and "no" are used to answer questions. If a negative is used in the question asked, a Japanese speaker is apt to answer "yes" to affirm the negative posed in the question. A native English speaker would generally answer "no" in the same circumstances to mean the very same thing that the native Japanese speaker would mean with the "yes" answer. For example, if asked, "You're not going to the store just now, are you?," a Japanese person would answer "yes" to mean they are not; Americans would usually answer "No, I'm not." Part of this is due to the difference in how the original question would be asked in the Japanese language ("are you" would not appear in Japanese).

Genetic counseling and evaluation for a traditional Japanese person can be, at the very least, baffling and confusing. Nondirective counseling would not be culturally correct for traditional Japanese persons. Such individuals may expect direct advice from the counselor on whether or not to undertake tests or treatment. Since the physician is expected to direct the care, he or she should formally authorize a referral to a genetic counselor and indicate clearly to the patient that this is being done. Furthermore, some genetic counseling involves no physical examination and no medicine; therefore, it may not be seen as meeting expectations of what is perceived to be Western-style health care.

Since genetic counseling and evaluation require the disclosure of very personal family information, it is imperative that genetics professionals assure the patient of privacy and gain his or her respect; otherwise, it may be hard to obtain accurate family history and other information. During the session, providers should maintain a respectful demeanor; for example a handshake is acceptable, but not a pat on the back, which would be too familiar.

Prenatal testing (i.e., amniocentesis or chorionic villus sampling) should be presented in the usual sensitive manner. Abortion can be considered as a possibility, since male infants are still highly prized and an abnormal male infant could bring embarrassment and shame to the family name. Adoption is still relatively uncommon, except among family members. Since artificial insemination by a donor may imply something "defective" or negative about the husband or question his masculinity and ability to preserve the family, it may not be a viable option for many women. However, there is a strong belief in family and, therefore, some stigma attached to not having one's "own" children. Consequently, artificial insemination may be more acceptable than adoption, especially if done within the family and with the assurance of privacy (i.e., done in an anonymous or coded manner). GIFT and in vitro fertilization may be more acceptable.

Issues of nonpaternity and paternity are almost nonexistent. However, outside influences are changing many traditional behaviors. Consanguinity appears to have existed before World War II and became taboo because of outside influences. But, again, this may be a nonissue, since whom one marries (a cousin, for example) may not be as important as compatibility and its implications for harmony.

A high literacy rate and a clear emphasis on education are common throughout modern Japanese society. Today, even rural areas have access to television and other means of communication. Scientific discoveries and new diagnostic techniques are known; therefore, patients understand the need for venipuncture, biopsies, and other methods of diagnostic specimen collection.

Events in the life cycle are viewed as transient, with an understanding of life's impermanence: individuals are born, live, die, and are reborn. Death is seen as a part of the cycle of life. The concept of brain death is new in Japan and not totally accepted. Aggressive life-saving procedures, therefore, are not seen as important as they are within the context of American culture and beliefs. Organ transplantation is difficult to accomplish since donations are almost nil. Individuals who want an organ transplant often go to Australia or another country where organs are more available.

Japanese families play an important role in life decisions. Usually, a diagnosis of cancer or similar life-shortening condition should not be initially shared with the patient. Instead, the provider should tell the family first, and they can decide if it is in the patient's best interest to know the diagnosis. Having a child diagnosed with a genetic syndrome may lead to stigmatization and even damage to the family name. Care must be taken not to lay blame that could harm the family. The family may refuse to grant permission to photograph an affected child, especially if the disorder is extremely deforming or embarrassing. Therefore, the maintenance of privacy and the intended use of the photograph only for medical research or education must be emphasized and observed. The use of such photographs for high school education or other lay activities would be inappropriate. Visual aids are acceptable, though providers should take the usual precautions against presenting pictures of very deforming disorders.

Children with severe disabilities may be hidden from view and omitted when giving the family history. Since World War II, there has been a gradual move toward educating handicapped children, but total mainstreaming has yet to be achieved. Children may be hidden in institutions. Counselors should be careful not to be judgmental.

Most resources for the family remain within the family. The family is involved in hospital care as much as are professional personnel. Outside resources may be neglected and the use of U.S. government aid viewed as a failure of the family.

The death of an individual and the request for an autopsy may be met with soft-spoken but firm resistance. The autopsy procedure represents a violation of the body and a terrible invasion of privacy. Grief is handled privately and stoically. Death is more accepted and may not be as traumatic an event as in Western culture.

CONCLUSION

Japanese culture is constantly changing. Japan's economic impact on the world has brought the nation not only affluence but also the influence of other cultures. For recent immigrants, the degree of acculturation will vary greatly, but Americans of Japanese origin are culturally more allied with their birth nation than with Japan. Before beginning the counseling session, the health care provider should try to ascertain the expectations of the individual couple and family and act appropriately. Not only is what is said important but also how it is said and what the listener perceives.

SUMMARY

—Inquire as to what the family religious background is. Try to determine the degree of Western acculturation. Assume a Western or American cultural orientation for third-, fourth-, and fifth-generation individuals, and treat them as Americans not as Japanese. It would be insulting to do otherwise.

—An introduction should include titles. Greet individuals as Mr. or Mrs. The family name is written first.

—Explain what will happen in the counseling session and explain the expectation that the patient will ask questions and participate in discussions. Patients may expect a full physical examination and treatment.

—Adoptions and autopsies are rare, as are organ transplantation donations.

—Assure the family of privacy and confidentiality.

—Explain the Western need for consent forms.

—Stress the importance of "no fault," especially with carrier testing.

—Establish rapport with the family by asking how they are, but remain formal.

—Allegiance to family is above the needs of the individual.

—Families may make major decisions. Allow an opportunity for this, if necessary. The family may need to consult family elders before making a decision.

—Inquire as to the patient's social support system.

—Avoid humor.

—Give thorough explanations; few questions may be asked.

—Photographs may be declined, especially if the child is deformed. The family may view the disability as shameful.

—A nod of the head indicates attentiveness, not necessarily agreement. "I understand" and "yes" do not always mean agreement.

REFERENCES

Cheng, L. R. 1990. Asian-American cultural perspectives on birth defects: Focus on cleft palate. *Cleft Palate Journal* 27:294–300.

Clark, M. M. 1983. Cultural context of medical practice. *Western Journal of Medicine* 139:806–10.

Creighton, M. R. 1990. Revisiting shame and guilt cultures: A forty-year pilgrimage. *Ethos* 18:279–307.

Hamilton, V. L., and Hagiwara, S. 1992. Roles, responsibilities, and accounts across cultures. *International Journal of Psychology* 27:157–79.

Haysaka, H., Ishii, H., Ambo, H., and Ohashi, H. 1991. The functions of "family" in health care systems: A health diary study in Japanese cities. *Tohoku Psychologia Folia* 50:62–68.

Herbig, P. A., and Miller, J. C. 1991. The effect of culture upon innovativeness: A comparison of the United States and Japan sourcing capabilities. *Journal of International Consumer Market* 3:7–54.

Koh, H. H., and Iwata, O. 1993. A cross-cultural study of socially appropriate behavior between Korean and Japanese undergraduates. *Psychologia* 36:185–91.

Locke, D. 1992. *Multicultural Understanding: A Comprehensive Model.* Newbury Park, Calif.: Sage.

Miron, G., and Katoda, H. 1991. Education for persons with handicaps in Japan, the U.S.A., and Sweden. *Scandinavian Journal of Educational Research* 35:163–78.

Reischauer, E. O., and Fairbank, J. K. 1989. *East Asia: Tradition and Transformation.* Boston: Houghton Mifflin.

Wu Dunn, S. Mizuku jizo. *New York Times,* 25 January 1996.

7

Culture of the Countries of Southeast Asia

Nancy L. Fisher, R.N., M.D., M.P.H., and
Lillian Lew, M.Ed., R.D.

Southeast Asia is a diverse geographic area consisting of Burma, Cambodia, Indonesia, Laos, Malaysia, the Philippines, Singapore, Thailand, and Vietnam. Since the newest and largest influx of immigrants to the United States in recent years are individuals from Laos, Cambodia, and Vietnam, this chapter will focus on the people from these three countries.

HISTORY AND MIGRATION

Laos is mostly covered by mountains. The majority of its diverse ethnic groups are Hmong ("free"), Mien ("people"), and lowland Lao. A country marked by constant struggle with neighboring Burma, Cambodia, and Thailand, it was colonized by France in 1893. Laos became an independent state in 1954 but civil strife continued. In the 1960s it became involved in the Vietnam War. The government collapsed in 1975 and reprisals were instituted against the Mien and Hmong, who had helped the U.S. military. Refugees fled across the Thai / Mekong border.

Vietnam has mixed terrain. The northern part is mountainous, while the southern part is flat, formed by the Mekong Delta. Its hot climate is ideal for growing rice, and the country is strategically located for trade. Recorded history goes back several thousand years. Despite domination by China, Japan, and France, Vietnam has maintained its identity. While the French brought medicine, education, and government, they caused severe economic and cultural upheaval. Both North and South Vietnam were opposed to French rule. Although the French were ousted, the fighting did not stop until the country was divided into a northern section, with Communist rule based in Hanoi, and a southern, non-Communist section. Reunification took place in 1956, but civil war erupted into a full-scale war by 1960. The Vietnam War forced more than one million people to seek asylum, and an estimated two million were killed. The well-educated, urban, middle-class professionals were the first to be airlifted out of the country to the United States or France. The second group of refugees were primarily relatives of the first. The "boat people" left in the late 1970s and early 1980s to escape "re-education" or more severe reprisals.

Cambodia is primarily a flat country. Its Khmer people date back almost two thousand years. Like Laos, it, too, has been in conflict with and dominated by Thailand, Vietnam, and France. Although Communism was suppressed in the country, the North Vietnamese did get a foothold. This action allowed the Cambodian Communists, the Khmer Rouge and Red Cambodians, to gain strength. In 1975, the Khmer Rouge leader, Pol Pot, defeated the North Vietnamese Communists and cleared Pnomh Penh of its total population. The region was renamed Kampuchea. The Khmer Rouge attempted to eradicate Western influence by killing the wealthy and educated. The killing decreased after the Vietnamese invasion of the country in 1978 as efforts were refocused. Only in 1979, as the Cambodian refugees began to escape across the Thai border, did the rest of the world learn of the genocide that left an estimated one to three million Cambodians dead.

Most refugees and survivors from these Southeast Asian countries have several things in common: displacement, loss of family, witnessing untold atrocities and hardships, and prolonged stays in refugee camps.

RELIGION

Buddhism, Confucianism, and Taoism, which may be perceived by Westerners as passive, have all influenced cultures in countries of Southeast Asia. Many people from Southeast Asia strive to live in harmony; direct confrontation is to be avoided. There is no requirement to believe in God, but instead to rely on personal responsibility for one's life. Many young Cambodian and Laotian males go to a local temple *(Wat)* for three months to become novice monks *(sangha)*.

The Buddhism practiced in Vietnam has quite different beliefs. Religion may be a mix of Brahmanism, Hinduism, animism, and spirit worship. There is a belief in spiritual and supernatural powers, and everything is believed to possess a soul. Many Vietnamese worship their ancestors. There is a strong belief in the power of all living creatures to change destiny.

The Laotian "soul" ceremony is performed at important occasions. The purpose is to make contact with the body spirits by calling them back to the body and thereby invoking their protective powers. The King of the souls resides in the head; therefore, touching the head is taboo and is believed to lead to bodily or mental dysfunction.

Religious life throughout Southeast Asia has also been influenced by Western religious beliefs. Catholicism influenced culture in Vietnam, and almost one-third of the early immigrants to the United States practiced that religion. Twenty-six percent of the Mien are Christian (Baptist). Some converted because it was rumored that conversion would permit entry into the United States, while others converted to help cure illness. Animism also has a strong influence. Many worship the Earth god, observe astrology and the twelve-year cycle marked by different animals.

FAMILY

The family is the center of culture and society of people from Southeast Asian countries. The immediate family includes the husband, wife, children, and sons' wives. The extended family includes close relatives and those sharing last names, as well as ancestors. The Hmong define family members to include individuals in their clan in the same community.

The husband is the principal provider and takes care of the family's interactions with people outside of the family. The wife is primarily responsible for the family's internal affairs. In many Vietnamese families, the wife has no status until she provides a son. Parental responsibilities extend more to children than to a spouse. Parents will make great personal sacrifices for the welfare of the family.

Infants are considered helpless, and preschool is the time to begin discipline. The Hmong may give children numbers, rather than names, until they are two years of age, to protect them from evil spirits. The Vietnamese dress infants in old clothes until one month of age to prevent spirits from being jealous of the child. If a Cambodian child becomes ill, the parents change the child's name, thereby confusing the spirits and, they hope, protecting the child. Children learn their role in the family in terms of the duties, obligations, and responsibilities they are assigned. In general, people from Southeast Asian countries adhere to their traditional child-rearing practices; aggression, irresponsible acts, and disobedience are punished.

Dependence on the social group is encouraged in families from the Southeast Asian region. Elderly people expect to live with the extended family. If they have no children of their own, they live with the extended family or an "adopted" family. Childbearing begins early, and having grandchildren by forty years of age is not uncommon. Once a grandparent, an individual is considered by the rest of the family to be elderly. Reverence and respect are given to the elders and ancestors. An individual's behavior reflects on the family and can cause either pride or shame to those both living and deceased.

Strong traditions and sense of familial security lend a sense of permanence overall. Life is considered to be a cycle of events—living and dying. Traditions may change, but only very slowly. Therefore, the sense of punctuality and time urgency varies greatly from that of Western cultures.

COMMUNICATION

Khmer is the official language of Cambodia, and has many dialects. Chinese and Cham are also spoken. The Khmer have a written language of sixty-six consonants and vowels. It is written from left to right and top to bottom.

The official language of Laos is Lao. It has written symbols based on Sanskrit and consists of fifty vowels and consonants. Mien has no written language, but records were written in Chinese characters. The Mien in the United States consist primarily of six groups, or clans, whose names begin with *Sae:* Saepharn, Saeteurn, Saelee, Saefong, Saeliaw, and Saechao. However, the spellings of these names may differ. The Hmong have few, if any, written historical records, but do have a written and oral language.

While French is the second language of Vietnam, Vietnamese has three primary dialects. The writing system is based on the Roman alphabet, with thirty consonants and vowels (see table 7.1).

It is important to note that many medical terms, especially in genetics,

Table 7.1. Languages and Dialects Common in Southeast Asian Countries

Country	Language	Dialect
Cambodia	Khmer	Khmer
		Teachiu (Chinese)
		Cham (Chom)
Laos	Lao	Hmong
		Lao
		Khmu
		Mien
		Tai
		Teachiu (Chinese)
Vietnam	Vietnamese	Bahnar
		Cantonese
		Cham
		Rhode
		Vietnamese

usually cannot be translated (e.g., *chromosome, karyotype, DNA,* and *gene*). Genetic professionals may need to explore lengthy but simple explanations. The label of Down syndrome may not exist but, for example, one woman, upon seeing a picture of a child with trisomy 21, revealed, "My brother has this."

Many individuals from the Southeast Asian region believe that the principal goal of language is to promote unity and harmony. Therefore, conversation may have shaded meanings, indirect intent, and numerous nonverbal cues. Social status, age, sex, and education may dictate the manner of address. People from Southeast Asia may use indirect eye contact or a bowed head when with people in authority. Eye contact or a nod of the head can mean "no" when the listener does not wish to offend. Nonverbal communication is paramount to interaction, and silence is valued. The latter is sometimes used to show respect and interest. If the person cannot accept the speaker's attitude or opinion, silence preserves harmony and peace.

Control of emotion is highly valued and should not be interpreted as stoic or uncaring. Similarly, any direct eye contact in interactions with strangers is not appropriate and is considered disrespectful to those in positions of authority. Smiling is the appropriate response to a compliment. A verbal "thank you" is unexpected and inappropriate.

Offensive gestures include: beckoning with an upturned finger (used to call animals); pointing (seen as aggressive or threatening); slapping on the back or stepping in front of someone; raising hands above someone; standing above someone; pointing or touching with the feet; and crossing the middle and index fingers for good luck (this is obscene). The Western gesture of waving good-bye is similar to that of beckoning. Public hand-holding is readily accepted between members of the same sex, but not between opposite sexes.

Since many Westerners do not speak Lao, Mien, Hmong, Vietnamese, or Cambodian, interpreters are often necessary in a genetic counseling session. It helps to choose an interpreter of the same ethnicity. The Southeast Asian countries have had many years of strife and war among themselves. A Vietnamese family may not trust a Cambodian person who speaks Vietnamese, and may withhold information or offer incorrect information. It is important to ask the interpreter how the family members should be addressed and what the family expects from the visit. Usually, older members are greeted before younger ones and males are greeted before females. The use of interpreters of the same sex as the patient avoids embarrassment and undue modesty. Such questions as date of last menstrual period (LMP) will be more readily answered with an interpreter of the same sex. Showing respect to the interpreter will encourage the patient and the family to trust that this interpreter can adequately convey their information and feelings. Children should not be seen as wiser than adults, so health care providers should not employ them as interpreters unless the family brings them for this specific purpose. Educating interpreters about genetic disease and the importance of obtaining accurate and complete family histories can make the medical encounter less stressful for all involved. The more the interpreter understands, the better the job he or she can do.

CULTURE

Calendars may vary among groups in Southeast Asia, as does the calculation of age. Many Vietnamese are considered one year old at birth. This can cause problems when plotting growth and development on Western standardized charts. Also, the age of new immigrants may be designated incorrectly. The strong tendency to avoid any conflict and seek asylum results in acceptance of whatever age an immigration official records upon entry into the United States. Also, in many cases, due to the lack of written records, the calculation of age has been tied to significant historical events, such as wars or floods. This is significant in referral for prenatal diagnosis, since an age difference of two to three years can greatly change the age-related risk of aneuploidy.

The definition of consanguinity varies. Many people from Southeast Asian countries accept that first cousins may marry if their last names are different. However, for others it is taboo for the younger sister's son to marry the older sister's daughter, even if the family name is not the same. However, it may be acceptable for the older sister's son to marry the younger sister's daughter.

Education is highly valued, and teachers have status and great social significance in many societies in Southeast Asia. By doing well in school, a child brings honor to the family. Other virtues revered are thrift, industry, patience, endurance, tolerance, and accommodation. Human suffering is considered a part of the natural order, so the individual must accept fate and show restraint. Grief is private.

BELIEFS ABOUT HEALTH

Each group has its own traditional beliefs about healing, but there are some commonalities. Illness falls into three categories: physical, metaphysical, and supernatural. Physical illness is caused by accidents or eating spoiled food. Recognized diseases include leprosy, tuberculosis, malaria, cholera, and hepatitis. Metaphysical illnesses may be caused by bad wind, an imbalance of hot/cold energy, an incorrect diet, or excessive emotion. Supernatural illness may be caused by the spirits or a loss of one's soul.

Metaphysical causes of illness are based on the principle of *yin* and *yang*, the Chinese dualistic philosophy consisting of two elements: one negative, dark, and feminine (yin), and the other positive, bright, and masculine (yang). The interactions of yin and yang are believed to influence the destinies of creatures and things. Illness and remedies are classified as either cold or hot. To have good health, one's yin/yang polarity must be balanced and in harmony. For example, if pregnancy is considered cold, treating it with a "cold" remedy such as vitamins would not restore balance. Diet must be balanced, including consumption of both cold and hot substances. However, the classification of what is cold or hot may differ among various ethnic groups.

It is believed that a major cause of supernatural illness is loss of soul. To have good health, all souls must be present in the body. Souls may be frightened away or shaken loose from the body. Surgery is seen as a loss of soul. Also, *any* loss of blood is associated with a shortened life span. At birth, one is given an allotment of blood, and its loss is viewed by some as irreversible.

Some believe that illness can be caused by bad spirits or even by offending a good spirit. Many Cambodians consider seizures to be not a physical problem, but rather possession by a spirit. Because of this, episodes may not be reported in family histories. A person who believes his or her illness is caused by the supernatural will not have confidence in Western medical practices, but may listen politely so as not to offend the genetic professional.

Remedies for pains and illnesses may vary from family to family and are passed on through an oral tradition. Health care providers include herbalists, Shamans, soul callers, Buddhist monks, pharmacists, and "injectionists." Few hospitals exist throughout this region, and those that do are concentrated in urban areas. Hospitals are often viewed as a place to go to die. Amulets are often worn. Knots in the string represent prayer, and some consider it a form of psychological violence to remove the amulets.

Pharmacists can diagnose and treat as they see fit. A person may go to the pharmacist and order any medicine. Many still obtain medicine through the mail or at local Southeast Asian–owned businesses. Injectionists are usually former army medics or nursing aides who establish a business to give medicine. They travel between villages, offering their services. The Mien have traditionally had older women with expertise in herbs who would prescribe treatments. The limited availability of the herbs in the United States has decreased their use.

The Mien use "Sar treatments" for illnesses attributed not to ancestors, but to hormonal imbalance. Tiger balm, lime or lemon juice, salt, ginger, mint, lemon grass, onion, and garlic are commonly used as treatments.

Dermabrasion is a common cure for "bad wind," a metaphysical illness caused by the invasion of "cold" into the body. This cold is believed to cause an imbalance between hot and cold in the body. Literally translated, dermabrasion means "rubbing of the skin"; it introduces heat into the body to "suck out the cold" and restore the body's balance. Dermabrasion consists of coining *(cao gio)* and spooning the skin, using the edge of a coin or spoon to rub the skin of the back in a linear fashion. It produces superficial bruises. Pinching *(bat gio)* is used for minor ailments and pain. Cupping *(giac)*, using a cup to create a vacuum with the skin over the forehead, is used to suck out pain. Pinching and scratching may be done over any affected area. White tape is also placed over places of pain. The treatment of last resort is burning; it is not unusual to see cigarette burns on an abdomen.

The Mien culture also employs healing ceremonies for spiritual causes of illnesses. *Sip mien* ceremonies encompass fourteen different protective and healing ceremonies. (*Mien* means ancestor spirits, and sip mien is performed to protect living family members.) Some ceremonies require a written record of the family's genealogy for as many as ten generations. *Phat* is a ceremony performed only by priests. It calls for the ancestor spirit rather than the afflicted. It is used for children suffering from soul fright, respiratory illnesses, sprains, or broken bones. Miens who converted to Christianity were required to destroy family records needed to perform phat and sip mien.

Belief in karma and fate is strong, and may extend to both living and dead family members. Saying "bad" things in genetic counseling may disturb the good aura of the family or ancestors. Because the majority of individuals are reactive rather than proactive, prenatal diagnosis may be viewed as not very important. In fact, the strong belief in fate makes predicting risk irrelevant. Since medical science cannot given an absolute answer, little value is placed on future investigation. Likewise, DNA storage or prenatal diagnosis is not a priority.

The fact that the cultural schema of anatomy, physiology, and scientific definition of illness differ or may not exist forms a major barrier not only to health care but also to genetic services. It is sometimes difficult to explain genes, chromosomes, and DNA, so counselors should keep explanations clear and simple. Diagrams and pictures may be helpful. However, for some individuals unfamiliar with the Western tradition of diagramming bodies without reference to the whole, the disembodied uterus and other parts of the anatomy in medical illustrations may be disconcerting or offensive.

Physical examination can pose problems. The head is the seat of the life essence; it is untouchable. The area between the waist and the knee is extremely private and personal. Pelvic examinations are often a fearful experience and may not be permitted until the second or third visit. Growth patterns of first-generation infants and children from Southeast Asian countries appear to differ from the standard of North American children. (Perhaps the growth charts reported by Baldwin and Sutherland [1988] would be more appropriate.)

Pregnancy is a special time, accompanied by various dietary and behavioral restrictions. Breaking taboos can be viewed as the cause of hyperactivity, developmental delay, or other congenital anomalies. Some individuals believe that viewing horror movies in early pregnancy or viewing pictures of a child with Down syndrome can cause the unborn child to have these or other health problems, so providers should ask permission to use medical illustrations. Using sharp instruments, such as scissors or a knife, may be believed to cause miscarriage or clefting of a lip or palate. During different gestational times in pregnancy, women may avoid being near doorways, specific appliances, or certain rooms to avoid spirits who may move throughout the house.

Some groups consider disability or mental retardation a stigma, while others believe in reincarnation and the obligation to care for the "special" person in this lifetime. They may have offended the "special" person in a previous lifetime and now they must atone for their previous behavior; if not, a future life can bring a worse fate. Moreover, others may believe the disability or problem is divine punishment for sins or transgressions of their ancestors, and they must atone.

Western medicine may be sought for specific remedies. Many Vietnamese people have a long history of French medical treatment and may accept Western medicine more readily. Many families rely on a blend of both medical systems. It is useful to inquire of families what they call a particular disorder, what they believe to be the cause and cure, and which treatments they have already sought.

IMPLICATIONS FOR GENETIC SERVICES

Health care providers should begin the session with a proper greeting, avoiding direct questions immediately. Standing or sitting higher than the family during the session is insulting. Providers should keep the session formal and avoid patting children on the head. Women usually do not shake hands with men, and younger people do not shake hands with elders. Direct physical contact should be avoided.

American English is highly ingrained with jargon and can indirectly lead to misunderstandings. Requesting the "Christian" name is inappropriate, as many families are not Christian. Using an interpreter may cause a session to be twice as long as usual, so providers should give the interpreter time to explain the sequence of the session to let the family know what to expect. (For example, many people expect to receive medication at the end of the session and may feel dissatisfied if they do not get it. Explaining the purpose of the visit should avoid such problems.) In fact, it is wise to decide before a session exactly what information is important to ascertain and how to best achieve this. Visual aids depicting chromosomes, genes, and other items are helpful, but providers should ask permission before showing pictures of any affected people. Questions should be directed to the appropriate individual, but without a prolonged gaze. Above all, politeness and tact will help the session move smoothly.

For a prenatal diagnosis counseling session, counselors should determine whether the pregnant woman's recorded or stated age is correct. "Mistakes" (such as in immigration records) have occurred and have radically altered the risk for age-related aneuploidy.

Consanguinity may become apparent only when drawing a pedigree. Review it with the family; sometimes an individual is placed twice in the pedigree without being identified. As in Western culture, the couple may be embarrassed to state that they have an "improper" marriage and may need to "save face" by avoiding this issue. One couple changed their names during immigration so that they would be permitted to marry. During a genetic counseling session they had to be assured of confidentiality before they would disclose this very pertinent information. (It was helpful to congratulate them on their cleverness.)

Many clients come to a genetic counseling session, understand the risks, and then refuse prenatal diagnostic procedures; part of having a choice is the ability to decline. However, others do not respond to nondirective counseling and wish to be told what to do by the physician, who is viewed as the authority figure. It is not uncommon for a physician or counselor to be asked directly what he or she would choose to do in a similar situation. Examples of actions and consequences may be a solution. The couple will need to know the heart complications, mental retardation, and other features of a chromosomal alteration. The counselor may need to explore how this will impact *their* family and community, besides revealing how Western culture views physically and mentally challenged individuals.

Clinics should not be scheduled on days that have cultural significance. The Vietnamese New Year is usually celebrated for several days and is called "Tet." The first day of the fifth month of the lunar calendar is the Cambodian and Laotian New Year; it usually falls in mid-April. Interpreters can advise on holidays that could affect the clinic schedule.

When drawing blood, microsamples are best for adults and children alike. It is believed that a person is given his or her lifetime supply of blood at birth, and blood loss is seen as detrimental, even when it is for medical purposes. Sometimes drawing blood and giving a pink drink can alleviate some individuals' hesitancy. Educating the patient about the reproduction of red blood cells every 120 days also helps to allay some fears. It is a good precaution to advise laboratories of the importance of handling blood samples carefully. Repeating laboratory tests is not a practical option, so providers should plan ahead.

Reproductive technologies may be less acceptable to Cambodians and Laotians with little exposure to Western medicine, but more acceptable to Vietnamese, who have had more exposure to Western medicine imported by the French. Abortion and artificial insemination by a donor are usually not sought, as they may be seen as interfering with fate, reincarnation, and harmony. Family planning, birth control pills, DepoProvera, and other means of birth control are chosen on an individual basis. Finances can constrain and affect not only health care but also family size. However, acculturation occurs at different levels and over different time spans. Amniocentesis may be accepted, because it conforms to societal reality and preserves harmony. Adoption out of the family may not be considered an option, because the individual is a product of all generations and is viewed as an integral part of a family. However, for couples with infertility problems, adoption may be acceptable. For many, the adoption of nieces, nephews, and close and distant cousins is one way of keeping the bloodline and family intact.

When explaining the cause of cleft lip and palate, spina bifida, and other conditions, providers should be sure to ask patients what they believe caused this, so that their concerns are better addressed. It is also wise to ask which treatments, if any, have already been sought. Some may be harmful to the unborn fetus. Nonpaternity is usually not an issue with the "older" generation. Tact and an indirect approach are recommended. Providers should listen, then address only those problems that may damage the affected individual. Trying to find a compromise to any area of disagreement is worthwhile, since the family will seek out a traditional healer if they are inappropriately handled. Whether the family members follow the recommendations for outside assistance will depend, in part, on how important they think the problem is and how they perceive the institutions and individuals providing care. Families usually consent to autopsies for a determination of the cause of death, as, for example, when poisons may be involved. However, if a child with multiple anomalies dies, death is viewed as an "answer," and no additional investigation is needed.

Illustrations from everyday life can help providers explain genetic issues, such as explaining risk in autosomal recessive disorders with a lottery system. For example, altered and unaltered genes can be represented by money: each parent gives the child a dime (an unaltered gene) or a penny (an altered gene). If the child receives two dimes (not affected), or a penny and a dime (carriers, but not affected), he or she is healthy. However, a problem will arise if the child receives two pennies (affected), as this is the least money one can "inherit." In this case, the child would have the disease. This example is useful for explaining situations after the diagnosis of an affected child.

The lottery can also be used to illustrate the concept of independent occurrence. In the lottery, the same numbers are used every week, regardless of whether they have been used previously. Because one number has been previously used does not mean that it cannot be used again, or not used again the next week. Similarly, this illustrates how the same genes can be used repeatedly, while the combination varies. On occasion, it is useful to relay this in story form, such that the good aura of the family is not disturbed.

Written handouts are helpful only if the patient can read—and only if a written language exists, which is not always the case. Patients should be asked in what language they wish the information. Sometimes English is appropriate, as sponsors can read and translate for families.

Providers should not take anything for granted. For example, wearing a white coat can be unsettling to the patient. White is a color of mourning and signifies bad luck, even death. Also, many people expect to receive medication at the closing of a session and may feel dissatisfied if they do not get it. Providers should explain this *before* the counseling session to avoid misunderstanding.

The patient's community is bonded not only in common culture but also in the shared experience of displacement from a native country and the consequent stresses. People rely on each other. Support groups are used within communities, but rarely outside. However, it is not insulting to suggest a support group, even if it is outside the patient's community.

In giving a family history, individuals are usually open and honest, and give what information they know. Some may refuse to give information because they believe it will have an impact on their public assistance (Medicaid). For this reason, mothers may state that they do not know the whereabouts of a child's father.

Finally, anecdotal evidence seems to indicate that a great variety of birth defects and genetic disorders occur in children and adults from Southeast Asian countries. However, hemoglobinopathies have a high prevalence. He-

Table 7.2. Incidence of Thalassemia in People of Southeast Asian Descent

Country	Alpha Carrier (%)	Beta Carrier	Hb E (%)	Hb E / Beta
Laos	40.0	Common	35–50	
Cambodia	Common	Common	35–50	
Vietnam	Common	Common	2–5	
Indonesia	0.5	Common	2–5	
Burma	10.5	Common	>10	Common
Malaysia	Common	Common	2–5	

Note: Glucose-6-phosphate dehydrogenase (G-6-PD) deficiency is common in all groups.

moglobin E and the beta and the alpha thalessemias are very common (table 7.2). Glucose-6-phosphate dehydrogenase (G-6-PD) is common enough that before the prescription of sulpha and other related drugs, screening should be considered.

CONCLUSION

Many immigrants have come to the United States and Canada not because they wished to leave their country but because they were forced to flee. The North American culture is strange and unfamiliar to them. Each individual will acquire acculturation in his or her own specific time frame. The population is diverse, with varying educational professional skills and economic skills. Like many new immigrants, they have been stereotyped and viewed with suspicion. North Americans who tend to see individuals from Asia as "all looking alike" will not get to know the true person, and health care providers must make sure not to miss the opportunity for appropriate genetic counseling. It is the health care provider's task to make genetic counseling as nonconfrontational as possible. Proper introduction into the community will also help in establishing rapport and trust.

SUMMARY

—If using an interpreter, discuss before the counseling session how to address the patients, their expectations, and their beliefs about Western medicine.
—Do not beckon individuals with the fingers. Assess the amount of eye contact and adjust it according to the patient's comfort level.

—Working with an interpreter will probably double the length of the appointment. Decide what is essential and appropriate to cover, and focus on these items first.

—In prenatal counseling, inquire as to the method of calculating the reported parental ages.

—Ascertain the level of acculturation. Individuals in the United States longer may be more familiar and comfortable with Western medicine.

—If blood tests are done, do not draw extra blood. Arrange for the use of microtubes, if possible.

—Never pat a child on the head.

—Respect the patient's right to refuse procedures. Do not assume that refusal indicates a lack of understanding.

—Ask permission to use visual aids.

—If the patient desires written handouts, provide them in his or her language.

—When using an interpreter, speak directly to the patient. Try to use interpreters of the same ethnicity and sex as the patient. Try to avoid using children as interpreters.

—Leave white coats at home!

—Learn about the community leaders and associations. Speak with them about establishing a clinic.

—For introductions, use last names and professional titles, if any.

—Ask open-ended questions rather than direct questions.

—Recommendations should be specific and short-term. Give careful consideration to the social impact of any recommendation. Work toward consensus within each family.

—Silence may be an indication of thoughtful pondering. Do not try to "fill up" the silence.

REFERENCES

Baldwin, L., and Sutherland, S. 1988. Growth patterns of first-generation Southeast Asian infants. *American Journal Disease of Children* 142:526–31.

Buckwald, D., et al. 1992. Use of traditional health practices by Southeast Asian refugees in primary care clinic. *Western Journal of Medicine* 156:507–11.

Dahlberg, K. 1980. Medical care of Cambodian refugees. *Journal of the American Medical Association* 243:1062–65.

Fisher, N. L. 1992. Ethnocultural approaches to genetics. *Pediatric Clinics of North America* 39:55–64.

Gilman, S. C., et al. 1992. Use of traditional and modern health services by Laotian refugees. *Western Journal of Medicine* 157:310–15.

Hoang, G. N., and Erickson, R. V. 1982. Guidelines for providing medical care to Southeast Asian refugees. *Journal of the American Medical Association* 248:710–14.

Kemp, C. 1985. Cambodian refugee health care beliefs and practices. *Journal of Community Health Nursing* 2:41–52.

Hollingsworth, A. O., Brown, L. P., and Broaten, D. A. 1980. The refugees and childbearing: What to expect. *RN* 43:45–48.

Lee, E. 1988. Cultural factors in working with Southeast Asian refugee adolescents. *Journal of Adolescence* 11:167–79.

Lew, L. S. 1989. *Understanding the Southeast Asian Health Care Consumer: Genetic Services for Underserved Populations.* National symposium, Arlington, Va.

———. 1990. Understanding the Southeast Asian health care consumer: Bridges and barriers. *Birth Defects* 26:147–54.

———. 1991. Elderly Cambodians in Long Beach: Creating cultural access to health care. *Journal of Cross-Cultural Gerontology* 6:199–203.

Locke, D. C. 1992. *Increasing Multicultural Understanding: A Comprehensive Model.* Newbury Park, Calif.: Sage Publications.

Minkler, D. H., et al. 1988. Family planning among Southeast Asian refugees. *Western Journal of Medicine* 148:349–54.

Muecke, M. A. 1983. In search of healers: Southeast Asian refugees in the American health care system. *Western Journal of Medicine* 139:835–39.

Schreiner, D. 1981. *SE Asian Folk Healing Practices/Child Abuse?* Indochinese Health Conference. Eugene, Ore. 18 September 1981.

Waxler-Morrison, N., Anderson, J., and Richardson, E. (eds.). 1990. *Cross-Cultural Caring.* Vancouver: University of British Columbia Press.

Yeatmin, G. W. 1980. *Cao gio* (coin rubbing): Vietnamese attitudes toward health care. *Journal of the American Medical Association* 244:2748–49.

8

Traditional Korean Culture

Sechin Cho, M.D.

Korea is a peninsula that borders on Manchuria and the Soviet Union to the north, faces China to the west across the Yellow Sea, and faces Japan to the east. The Korean peninsula and its adjacent islands cover an area of 221,362 square kilometers, which is about the same size as Great Britain. Korea has been divided into two halves since the end of World War II in 1945. South Korea has a population of approximately 40 million, and North Korea, 20 million.

The terrain of the eastern Korean peninsula is rugged and mountainous. The western part has many large rivers and rich, arable land. Korea enjoys a temperate climate with four distinct seasons: spring, summer, autumn, and winter.

HISTORY

It is believed that the history of the Korean people began about five thousand years ago with the influx of Mongolian tribes into the Korean peninsula. The ancient Korean peoples were heavily influenced by the Chinese who came to inhabit their lands. These invaders were finally driven from the Korean peninsula in A.D. 313, but they left a lasting imprint on the Korean culture.

According to ancient history, a god resembling a bear came down from heaven and settled on top of Taebeak Mountain, which lies in the northern part of the Korean peninsula. The god transformed a bear from earth into a woman and married her. They bore a son named Tangun, who, in B.C. 2333, founded Korea.

Around the first century B.C., Korea was divided into small kingdoms. The kingdom of Koguryo (B.C. 73–A.D. 668) was located in the northern half of the Korean peninsula and part of what is now Manchuria. The kingdom of Paeckche (B.C. 18–A.D. 668) lay in the southwestern part of the peninsula. It had very active trading and open communication with Japan. The people in this region first introduced Buddhism and the scripture to Japan in A.D. 550. The kingdom of Silla (B.C. 57–A.D. 668) was, in the beginning, the smallest of the three kingdoms. Later, it conquered Koguryo and Paeckche and unified as Korea.

The unified Silla Dynasty (668–936) witnessed the birth of the Golden Age of art and culture. Due to internal conflict and political corruption, the kingdom surrendered without resistance to the new leader of an opposition movement, Wang Kon.

Wang Kon, the first king of the new dynasty, established the Koryo period (918–1392). Wang Kon was a devout Buddhist. Therefore, Buddhism was a strong spiritual force during this period. Even though Confucianism had come to Korea during the period of the three kingdoms, it did not begin to gain influence until the end of the Koryo Dynasty. The current name Korea originated during the Koryo Dynasty. The Koryo Dynasty suffered as a result of the foreign invasion and domination. The eleventh and twelfth centuries were marked by sporadic clashes with various Chinese states. In 1231, Korea was invaded by Mongolians, whose domination followed until the demise of the dynasty.

General Yi Songgye, who achieved a distinguished military career while fighting Mongolian and Japanese invaders, toppled the Koryo Dynasty and founded a new dynasty, named Choson, or Yi dynasty (1392–1910). The rigid and literal application of Confucian doctrine dominated during the Yi Dynasty. The history of the Choson dynasty was as turbulent as that of the Koryo period. The country was invaded by Toyotomi Hideyoshi's Japanese military forces in 1592. Korea suffered from two further Manchu invasions, in 1627 and 1636.

As the result of foreign invasions, Korea adopted an isolationist policy and became known as the "hermit kingdom." By the early nineteenth century, Western traders and missionaries had tried to open Korea. In 1876, the country was open to Japan, followed by trade agreements with the United States, Russia, France, and Great Britain during the 1880s.

After the Sino-Japanese War (1894–95) and the Russo-Japanese War (1904–05), Korea was colonized by Japan in 1910. For thirty-six years, Korea was ruled by an oppressive colonial Japanese government and exploited for natural resources, living space, and labor. Unfortunately, the Japanese role during this period was not a benevolent one. It left a legacy of distrust and dislike between the two peoples. Anti-Japanese feelings are still very strong in Korea. Korea was again liberated from Japanese colonialism at the end of World War II (1945).

Between 1945 and 1948, the peninsula was under U.S. occupation in the south and Soviet occupation in the north. At that time, Korea was divided by the thirty-eighth parallel. On August 15, 1948, the Republic of Korea was formally established, with Syngman Rhee as the first president. And, on September 9, 1948, the Democratic People's Republic of Korea was proclaimed by Premier Kim Ilsung. On June 25, 1950, seventy thousand North Korean Communist military forces invaded South Korea and the Korean War began. This bitter war, which caused the sacrifice of many lives and much property, ended on July 27, 1953. Today, the South Korean democratic government is formed by free election.

RELIGION

It is believed that Buddhism first came to Korea in A.D. 372, when a Chinese king sent a group of Indian Buddhist monks to Koguryo. In 550, the kingdom of the Paeckche sent a Buddhist scripture and a golden image of Buddha to King Kimmei in the Japanese islands. Buddhism has, for centuries, played a great role in the development of art, architecture, literature, and performing arts.

Confucianism came to Korea from China before the introduction of Buddhism in 372. Confucianism dictated a system of education, ceremony, and civil administration as expressed by Confucius in his writings. The five codes of Confucius became the traditional way of behavior in Korean society. The codes suggest that there is justice between rulers and subjects, affection between father and son, prudence between husband and wife, order between old and young, and trust between friends. These codes even influence the form of address in the Korean language, which is structured in accordance with age, rank, and social position in writing or conversation.

During the Choson Dynasty (1392–1910), Confucianism became the official philosophy of the country. Now there are about 4.8 million Confucian converts, 12,000 monks, and 256 shrines.

The Koreans take pride in the largest Protestant population in Asia, with more than 6 million churchgoers and some 20,000 Korean clergy. The first two Protestant missionaries to set foot on Korean soil were Karl Kutzlaf of Germany in 1832 and R. J. Thomas of Scotland in 1865. The largest single denomination is Presbyterian, with 2.2 million members. Methodists have a following of 1.4 million. The Catholic Church was introduced by a Korean diplomat named Lee Sunghun, who was baptized by an Italian missionary in Beijing in 1873. Today, there are 1 million Catholics, 4,000 priests, and 500 Catholic churches.

Of the many other religious beliefs in Korea today, Chondogyo is unique and was established and founded in Korea. It is a very nationalistic religion for the people, allowing them to regain their Korean identity and revolt against alien religions, such as Buddhism, Confucianism, and Christianity. This sect claims 825,000 followers, 1,700 priests, and 140 churches.

Islam was first introduced to Korea by Turkish soldiers in Korea during the Korean War in 1955. There are 20,000 Korean Muslims today.

COMMUNICATION

In the sixth century, a scholar named Solchong invented the Idu form of writing, which translates Chinese characters into Korean vernacular. In 1145, *Samguk-sagi,* an early Korean history book based on old documents and Chinese sources, was written by the scholar Kim Pusik (1075–1151).

The most remarkable development in the Choson period was the invention of the Korean alphabet called *Hangul,* in 1446, by King Sejong. This writing system consists of fourteen consonants and ten vowels. It was designed on the basis of phonetic principles. It is unique; there is no relationship with Chinese or Japanese characters. The alphabet has an internal logic and the consistency makes it very easy to learn.

Koreans have three common forms of address: formal polite, informal polite, and informal. These forms are primarily indicated by specific group ending and choice of verb ending, depending on the perceived relationship among the people speaking. Status is conferred in Korea by sex, age, education, professional position, wealth, and relationship. Choosing the proper form of address is quite important to Koreans. Too low a form of address is considered insulting, while too high an address would be considered pandering on the part of the speaker.

FAMILY

Korean family life is closely knit among parents and children, brothers and sisters, and their spouses. The birth of a son is an occasion for great joy, more so than that of a daughter. The oldest son, as heir to the family name, is treated specially. He inherits most of the family property and, in turn, is expected to support his parents in their old age. If there is no son in the family, one might be adopted to fill the role of the first-born son. Often, the adoptee is a son-in-law, or brother's son, so that the family name is preserved.

Children, especially males, are pampered and not really disciplined until they reach school age. Children under age six, therefore, are somewhat fussy, noisy, disruptive, and rarely disciplined to the Western eye. Once children are of school age, they are subjected to rigorous discipline, a heavy work load, and close supervision.

Korean age does not represent completed years. The Korean baby is considered to be one year old on the day he or she is born. On the first birthday, a baby becomes two years old.

The celebration of birthdays has always been an important event for Koreans. Koreans celebrate one hundred days after the birth of a child, a very special event. The specific reason for the celebration is not known. However, it is believed that a child who survives the first hundred days is likely to survive to adulthood. Two other significant birthdays are the first birthday and the sixty-first birthday, celebrated with a traditional feast and gift-giving.

Marriages used to be arranged by parents through a go-between, or professional matchmaker. Courtship, therefore, was not customarily practiced in Korea. There is a noticeable change among educated people these days, however.

Consummating arranged marriages requires long, tedious formal steps. For example, the matchmaker must supply each side with a description of the person in question, as well as a family background. Consanguineous marriage is not permitted in Korea. A family history of a birth defect or genetic disorder is taboo and plays a very significant negative role in consummating marriages. Any family history of birth defects, mental retardation, and significant genetic disorders is omitted or hidden. Therefore, a family may consent to carrier testing only reluctantly, if at all. Stigmatization of women regarding X-linked recessive disorders can lead to familial stress and, in some cases, dissolution of marriages.

CULTURE

Ethnically, Korea is the most uniform country in the world. It is populated almost exclusively by a single ethnic group, the Han. All speak the Ural-Altaic language.

The most important factor in Korean history is its geographic location. China to the west and Japan to the east have fought many wars with each other and against Korea. This has led to the Korean peninsula's often being invaded and conquered, thus being heavily influenced by its two larger neighbors. Before the modern era, China was the most powerful influence in Korea, as exemplified in traditional Korean art.

Supposedly, the word *Shamanism* (*mudang* in Korean) may have originated from Siberian tribes. Shamanism is based on the belief that the visible world is pervaded by invisible forces or spirits that affect the lives of the living. The mudang performs magical rituals and plays the role of prophet or fortune teller. Shamanism has been ingrained in the minds of Koreans and informs the country's art, literature, music, and dance.

Despite heavy influence from Western cultures, some of the centuries-old values and customs are still preserved in modern Korea. The five codes of Confucius still govern the traditional home life. This can be seen in the respect one gives to elders. Drinking, smoking, singing, loud talking, or quarreling is not permitted in an elder's presence. Koreans remove their shoes when entering a home, many restaurants, and rooms in Korean-style inns.

Korea has two major traditional holidays that are celebrated throughout the country: Lunar New Year, which occurs between late January and the end of February, and Chusok, which occurs between late August and early October. Koreans wear traditional dress, *hanbok,* on Lunar New Year and Chusok. The basic costume for the Korean woman consists of a long, full skirt and a short jacket. The color combination is exquisite, utilizing many different-colored stripes. Most Korean women prefer the traditional costume to Western dress. However, this is not true for the Korean man, who prefers a Western business suit except for very special occasions, such as holidays and special ceremonies. Many elderly gentlemen still wear the traditional male Korean garment.

Most Korean dishes are grilled or sauteed. Rice is the most common staple diet among Koreans. Korean cuisine is very spicy and seasoned with garlic, onion, ginger, and red pepper. Notable Korean dishes are kimchi, bulgogi, kalbi, and bibimpap. Kimchi, which is made from cucumbers, radishes, carrots, greens, and other Chinese cabbages, is very hot and spicy. Bulgogi is thinly sliced, marinated beef that it is cooked on a cone of iron that is heated from inside. Kalbi is marinated beef short ribs baked at a low temperature for a long time until extremely tender. Bibimpap is a single ball of rice mixed with various condiments.

Touching among men and women is common and permissible in the Korean culture. Korean adolescent schoolgirls have close physical contact. They work hand-in-hand and arm-in-arm. The schoolgirls display the most extreme form of public physical contact among Koreans, but among almost all sex and age groups, touching is far more common than in most Western countries. Almost all such contact is intersexual and interfamilial. Adolescent boys and girls walking hand-in-hand or arm-in-arm are far more often brothers and sisters than lovers. In recent years, this has changed somewhat.

Westerners shake hands on meeting or departing, but Koreans bow in similar situations. In modern Korea, bowing and hand-shaking are practiced simultaneously. Korean women are less likely than Korean men to shake hands.

Unlike in the Western culture, gifts are received with formal and solemn thanks. However, it is not expected for the recipient to open the present or comment on it. Only when the recipient returns home, or the guests have gone, is the gift opened. The difference between a gift and a bribe is somewhat unclear in the Korean culture. On special occasions, it is customary that people of the lower pecking order give gifts to those of higher rank. Gifts are also given to those people with whom a person or organization has regular or special dealings. In Korean custom, such gifts are tokens of a special relationship and are not bribes. While gift-giving can be used to ensure a mutually favorable relationship, it is not intended to be used for special treatment.

Koreans think it impolite to say "no" bluntly in most situations. Often, they go to great lengths to avoid a blunt negative response, especially when dealing with a person of a higher social status, such as a physician. Other improprieties include sitting on the edge of a desk while addressing an audience, crossing one's arms on the chest while talking to elders, asking for a match or other service from an older person, putting one's hands on one's jaw during a conversation, and crossing one's legs on a sofa or chair in the presence of an elder (in most cases, a young person puts his hands together on his legs in front of an elder or superior).

BELIEFS ABOUT HEALTH

Koreans have developed a practice that is believed to improve pregnancy outcomes. They call it *Taegyo,* which translates as "fetal education." Once a pregnancy is confirmed, the woman is advised not to wash her hair during the ninth month of pregnancy, not to climb rocks or high places, not to drink alcoholic beverages, not to carry heavy loads, and not to consume grains other than rice. A second set of teachings dictates that a pregnant woman should not talk too much, place herself in situations that might surprise or frighten her, or cry. A third set of teachings advises pregnant women to avoid any occasion that might result in a fall. A fourth set of teachings urges pregnant women to sit down silently to meditate, to speak only beautiful words, to recite classic poems, and to listen to beautiful music. At the same time, the woman is encouraged not to listen to any complaints, not to see bad things, and not to harbor evil thoughts. Finally, sexual intercourse during the last part of pregnancy is prohibited. Women are told that, if they continue sexual intercourse, the newborn infant will die or be born prematurely.

Modern medical practice coexists with herbal medicine, folk practice, and psychic healing in Korea. Western medicine was introduced at the end of the nineteenth century to Korea by physician missionaries. Until that time, medical care for Koreans had depended on herbal medicines or care from an Oriental medicine doctor. In a short span of one hundred years, modern medicine in Korea has developed into world-class quality.

Medical school training consists of a two-year premedical course and four years of medical school. Medical school graduates undergo vigorous internship and residency, very similar to that in the United States. The public health system is well organized, and a public health center is available in every Korean city or county. The public health system concentrates on sanitation and the prevention of illness, and provides maternal/child health care and family planning. Koreans are very familiar with Western medicine, and it is the first choice when one becomes ill.

Even within the clinical setting, however, some differences prevail. For example, it is customary not to tell the patient of a fatal or incurable diagnosis. This information is communicated to the head of the family or the custodian of the child. Also, there is no fourth floor in hospital buildings and some hotels because the Korean words for the number *four* and *death* have the same sound.

Views on disability are tied to education, which in Korean culture is highly valued. Advancement in school is competitive, and tests not only include academic subjects, but greater than 50 percent may include some physical skill. Children with disabilities cannot fully compete. However, exceptions in society are made for individuals handicapped as a result of a war injury.

IMPLICATIONS FOR GENETIC SERVICES

When a health care professional interviews a Korean patient, it is very helpful to show respect to the interviewee, particularly to the oldest person. When a Korean person is not familiar with the English language, it is highly desirable to have an interpreter. A Korean family generally has very good pedigree information and is very family oriented. However, the history of genetic disease, mental retardation, and birth defects is not customarily conveyed to strangers. Therefore, practitioners will have the best success in obtaining information if an interpreter is secured from among family members.

Most well-established families have written pedigrees. In some cases, a pedigree will go back as far as seven hundred years. It has very good information on male family members, but little information on females. Koreans seldom have consanguineous marriage, and legally one cannot marry someone with the same last name. Nonpaternity rarely occurs. Common Korean surnames, such as Kim, Lee, Park, Chang, Choi, Han, and Cho, have several branches within the same surname.

Picture taking is not well accepted by Korean patients. If given a good explanation and reason for the request, however, the patient will usually agree. Blood drawing is also unpopular among Korean patients, but again if the patient understands the reason for the procedure, there should be no major problem.

The Korean patient has a tendency to trust male physicians more than female physicians. This gender bias has existed for a long time, and may require many more years until a female physician is treated on equal terms.

In the chart or any medical documents, one's name should not be written in red. The Korean patient may interpret this as a desire for death, since names are written in red ink on death certificates. If at all possible, admissions on the fourth floor and room numbers with the number four should be avoided.

The concept of written informed consent is foreign to the Korean patient. Korean doctors exercised authority over patients for many years. Therefore, a patient accepts the doctor's authority and trusts him or her. When a Korean patient is approached to sign an informed consent, he or she may become suspicious of the physician's ability to perform that particular procedure. Therefore, it is necessary to inform a Korean patient of the Western practice of obtaining informed consent.

The incidence of malpractice litigation is minimal in Korea. When treatment options include either an invasive procedure or medical treatment, Koreans tend to choose the noninvasive form of treatment and rely on fate.

Autopsy, DNA storage, and other tests for future planning may be irrelevant. Most Koreans want to die at home, and believe that in order to make the difficult journey to the next world they need valuable gifts, money, and other items for the trip. An autopsy would greatly handicap the person making this "journey." Individuals are buried on the third or fifth day after death. As one's status in society increases, the longer the wait to the funeral.

Genetic epidemiology has not been completely studied in Korea. In twenty-four hundred autopsies, including all age groups, congenital malformations were recorded as the cause of death in 4.4 percent of cases.

In the age group of 0 to 4 years, congenital malformation was reported as the cause of death in 10 percent of autopsy cases. The most common congenital malformation was cardiovascular malformation, followed by abnormalities of the central nervous system, vascular system, gastrointestinal system, oral cavity, and musculoskeletal system. Of the cardiovascular malformation group, ventricle septal defect was most common, representing 34.6 percent of congenital heart disease, tetralogy of Fallot (21.2 percent), atresia (18.1 percent), and atrial septal defect (7.4 percent). Of the gastrointestinal system malformations, intestinal stenosis / atresia was the most common, followed by imperforate anus, pyloric stenosis, intestinal stenosis or atresia, and biliary atresia. Among central nervous system malformations, meningomyelocele was the most common, followed by anencephaly, encephalocele, hydrocephalus, and holoprosencephaly.

The following chromosome abnormalities have been reported among Koreans: trisomy 21, trisomy 18, trisomy 13, trisomy 8, partial trisomy 10, monosomy 21, triploidy, 47 XXY, 45 X, 47 XXX, 47 XYY, fragile X chromosome, 2q-, 4q-, 5p-, 9p-, 13q-, 14p-, 18p-, 18q-, ring chromosome 18, 21q-.

Inborn errors of metabolism were studied vigorously during the 1980s in Korea. Documented inborn errors of metabolism include phenylketonuria, albinism, glycogen storage disease, Gaucher disease, Niemann-Pick disease, mucopolysaccharidosis, Wilson disease, congenital adrenal hyperplasia, methylmalonic acidemia, cystinuria, ornithine transcarbamylase (OTC) deficiency, homocystinuria, citrullinemia, Lesch-Nyhan syndrome, hyperoxaluria, mucolipidosis, metachromatic leukodystrophy, adrenoleukodystrophy, and Menkes disease. Among these, Wilson disease, glycogen storage disease, and congenital adrenal hyperplasia seem to be the most common. Most recently, the author discovered two cases of tetrahydrobiopterin synthetase deficiency. As diagnostic skills and laboratory facilities are improved, more reported cases of previously undiscovered inborn errors of metabolism will be identified. However, mental retardation or birth defects in a child are still considered by many to be associated with family shame or guilt. These problems are often blamed on the mother and are seen as a curse on her.

Prenatal diagnosis (e.g., amniocentesis, chorionic villus sampling) is well accepted among Koreans. Because they prefer to have male infants, it is very important to emphasize that the test is not designed to look for fetal sex, unless it is indicated for a sex-linked disorder. Fetal sexing in Korea is illegal. Since Koreans are heavily influenced by the teachings of Buddhism and Confucianism, the termination of a pregnancy does not invite the social discords witnessed in the United States.

Korea has a very successful family planning program, supported by an extensive public education program. Two children within one family is considered ideal. However, in discussing family planning options, providers should remember that some individuals may object to contraceptives because of religious beliefs. Artificial insemination by donor has been accepted on a small scale. Adoption outside the family is a foreign concept. Adoption *within* the family is done to continue the family name. For example, if the eldest son has no son, adoption of his brother's son may occur. Adoption outside the family occurs in small numbers, but may increase to stem the number of children being adopted outside of the country.

Korean patients look forward to having recommendations from the physician. Even in genetic counseling, Korean patients dislike nondirective counseling. They believe that they come to the genetic center to receive the best recommendation rather than to be informed of available options, which would leave them with the burden of making a decision. Therefore, in some cases, directive genetic counseling may be requested. Families look for internal support during crisis. Stress is not an acceptable reason for referral to a psychologist or psychiatrist. The latter are reserved for flagrant mental illness.

CONCLUSION

Despite the invasion of their geographical neighboring countries and influx of Westerners, Koreans have maintained their own customs and beliefs. Although more widely settled throughout the United States in comparison to other Asian groups, the Korean family is still a mainstay of support. After overcoming the stresses and limitations of new immigrants, Koreans are highly educated and entrepreneureal. As with other new immigrants, acculturation crises and intragenerational conflicts cause family stress. The likelihood of encountering an individual whose beliefs are not purely "traditionally" non-Western makes it imperative that the counselor listen closely to those seeking evaluation and counseling.

SUMMARY

—Greet males before females and shake hands only with males.

—Patients may feel it is important not to say "no" and will go to great lengths to avoid such responses with persons of higher social status.

—Do not stand above patients, sit on a desk, cross legs, or fold arms across chest. These gestures are considered impolite.

—Age is calculated differently. A child is two on the first birthday. This is important for advanced maternal age counseling and also in plotting growth and development on standardized charts.

—Marriages may still be arranged, so carrier testing and history of mental retardation and birth defects may be omitted or hidden.

—Do not write or draw with a red pencil. Do not use room four for counseling.

—Discuss the fact that prenatal testing is not done for the primary purpose of fetal sexing.

—Whenever possible, use family members as interpreters. One is usually more likely to receive "private" information during a family history this way.

—Photos are not well accepted, unless there is a strong medical concern.

—Do not expect immediate consent for blood drawing or skin biopsy. Reasons for these tests should be thoroughly explained.

—Explain the necessity for written consents. Otherwise, the consent process may raise doubts about the physician's ability.

—Use male counselors or geneticists whenever possible.

—Explain expectations of the counseling session first, since the patient may expect direct counseling and advice.

—Prenatal diagnostic testing, such as amniocentesis, chorionic villus sampling, and percutaneous umbilical blood sampling, may be declined because of the preference for noninvasive tests and belief in fate.

—Give bad news to the head of the family or the custodian of the child.

REFERENCES

Hyun, P. 1984. *Koreanna*. Republic of Korea: Korea Britannica Corporation.

Kim, K. T. 1991. *Korean History through Folklores*. Seoul: Hyum Fum Sa.

Steenson, G. 1987. *Coping with Korea*. New York: Basil-Blackwell.

Yang, S. M. 1991. *Korean Custom and Etiquette*. Seoul: Mon Yang Gak.

Personal communications with Drs. G. Chi, Ki Bok Kim, Dong H. Lee, and Hyung R. Moon in Seoul, Korea, 1995.

9

Traditional Asian Indian Culture

Shivanand R. Patil, Ph.D., and
Nancy L. Fisher, R.N., M.D., M.P.H.

The term *Asian Indian* is used to refer to individuals whose cultural origins include India, Pakistan, Bangladesh, Nepal, and Sri Lanka. Although these areas were all at one time under British rule, Asian Indians represent a socially and culturally diverse group. This chapter focuses primarily on the practices and beliefs common to many individuals in India. The information here is by no means to be considered a complete review of traditional beliefs. It is merely a glimpse at various activities of societies of diverse peoples. Furthermore, with the acceleration of trade and immigration in recent decades, traditional practices have loosened their hold, particularly in urban areas.

India is nearly one-third the size of the United States and has a population of 850 million people. The population density is 658 per square mile. India became a secular democracy after gaining its independence from Great Britain in 1947. The people of India live in deserts, high mountains, plains, tropical lowlands, and jungles. The terrain of India is as diverse as its people.

Hindi, the official language of India, is spoken by 30 percent of the population—primarily those living in the northern part of the country. English (associate official language) is spoken by only 3 percent, but it is important in government, education, and science. India's state boundaries are drawn largely along linguistic lines and the constitution recognizes fourteen other regional languages, even though more than two hundred languages are actually spoken. The major religion is Hinduism. About 83 percent of the population consider themselves Hindu, 12 percent Muslim, 3 percent Christian, 2 percent Sikh, 0.7 percent Buddhist, and about 0.5 percent Jain. The literacy level is approximately 36 percent. Over 70 percent of the population belongs to the ethnic group Indo-Aryan, and 25 percent are Dravidian. Mongol and other groups comprise approximately 3 percent of the populace. Farming is done by three-quarters of the population, but economic opportunities have spurred migration to the cities. Before 1950, the life expectancy was thirty-two years; now it is fifty-three years, with men living longer than women.

Most of Pakistan has cold winters and hot summers. The Himalayas and the Hindu Kush mountains in the north contain the highest peaks in the world. The official language of Pakistan is Urdu, but as in India, English is in general use in government, military, business, and higher education. Urdu is the native tongue of only about 10 percent of the population; Punjabi is spoken by over 60 percent, Sindhi by about 12 percent, Pakhtu by about 11 percent, Baluchi and Brahui by about 4 percent each. The nation is at least 98 percent Muslim, of which about 70 percent are Sunni; the remainder are Shiite, many of whom are Ismaili. Three-quarters of the populace live in rural areas, with an economy based on agriculture. The population is estimated at over 113 million, with a density of 335 per square mile.

Bangladesh (formerly East Pakistan) is surrounded primarily by India. The low-lying land is subjected to tropical monsoons, flooding, and famine. The major language is Bangla. The population is estimated at 118 million, and, at 3,028 per square mile, is the highest density in the world. More than 80 percent of the population practice Islam as their religion.

MIGRATION

Many Asian Indians immigrated to other countries in the British Empire to further their education and economic status. According to a U.S. Immigration and Naturalization report, 13 percent of the 130,000 Asian Indians entering the United States between 1820 and 1976 arrived before 1965. Exclusion laws passed in 1910, 1917, and 1923 virtually halted Asian Indian immigration for decades. Relaxation of the Asian quota in 1946 allowed limited immigration. In 1965, the immigration law eliminated national quotas, thereby dramatically increasing the number of Asians eligible to enter the country. Immigration to the United States has steadily grown since the 1960s. Many Asian Indians came to the United States to attend universities and did not need to be sponsored by relatives. The majority are first-generation, but an increasing number are North-American born. Many individuals are from urban centers and are well educated. By the 1990 U.S. Census, the Asian Indian population was 815,447, dispersed throughout the United States, except for concentrations in California of Sikh farmers in Yuba City and Gujaratis in San Francisco.

RELIGION

The most common religious groups among Asian Indians in North America are Hindus, Muslims, and Sikhs. These religions impose a structure on society and family life.

Hinduism

Hinduism denotes a diverse pattern of beliefs that include religion, attitudes toward life, and social behavior. There are various gods, styles of dress, worship, and eating habits. Beliefs are written in sacred scripture. Beef is strongly prohibited, and the cow is sacred, probably originating from its central role in agricultural life. Cow dung is used as fuel for daily cooking and for fertilizing the crops. Milk is a valued food for babies and youngsters. It is also used in making yogurt and butter, which play a major role in the vegetarian diet as well as religious ceremonies. Cows produce bulls and oxen, which are used to plow the fields. If beef could be eaten, there would not be enough cows to fulfill these other essential functions.

Hindus believe that life is a circle, continuous without beginning or end. Good fortune in this life depends on the behavior in a former life, according to the law of Karma. Each member is born into a caste, which has rules and regulations about who may cook and what foods are eaten.

Hindus attach importance to omens and luck. There is a strong belief in astrology, and individuals may have a fatalistic attitude. They believe that there are superior and inferior body parts: the left hand, left foot, and genitalia are inferior. It is considered bad luck if a person enters the house of a Hindu with the left foot first. A left-handed physician needs to mention this at the beginning of the patient visit.

Contraception is frowned upon and procreation desired. The family is the decision-maker. Abortion is a mild taboo (relating to the belief in the sanctity of life), and sex education is done in the home, female to female, male to male. During menstruation, sex and prayers are avoided. Child marriages do happen, though not legally. The sexes are segregated, and common-law marriages, courtship, and homosexuality are forbidden.

Bereavement is conducted within the family. Depending on the region, the funeral is followed by cremation, not burial. For the next three days, the family gathers at the home of the deceased and discusses the deceased and other deceased individuals. Meals are provided by the family. On the third day, relatives and friends congregate as an expression of sympathy. For the next ten days, women and men do not work but go to console the bereaved. On the tenth day, bereavement is closed. After that, the day of death is celebrated annually.

In contrast, until recently, birthdays were not celebrated. When a child is born, the mother may stay at home for forty days and is supported by female relatives. During labor, women may be encouraged to express feelings. A traditional birth ceremony may take place before the umbilical cord is cut, and approximately ten days later there is a naming ceremony.

At puberty, Brahman males have a ceremony where a sacred thread is tied across the shoulder and around the waist for the rest of his life.

Hindu women celebrate Brother's Day and Husband's Day. On the latter, women pray for a long life for their husbands. The Hindu Festival of Lights, or Diwali, is celebrated in October or November, according to a lunar calendar. Diwali has different connotations in the various regions of India. In some areas Diwali is a renewal of life. Holi is a spring festival celebrated in a variety of ways throughout India in February or March by people throwing colored water or colored powder on each other.

Islam

Muslims are individuals who submit to the will of Allah. The word *Allah* is Arabic for "God," and Muslims do not like it to be translated to avoid misinterpretation. Muslims reject all other gods and follow the teachings revealed by Muhammad, which are contained in the Koran.

Islam is based on five principles that encourage generosity, fairness, respect, and honesty:

1. The belief in Allah and his messenger Muhammad, to whom he revealed the Holy Qur'an (Koran).

2. Prayer five times a day, facing the direction of Holy Mosque at Mecca (namoz). Men and women are separated.

3. Fasting for one lunar month of the Islamic calendar every year (Ramadan).

4. Compulsory contributions to benefit the needy. Once a year, 2.5 percent of the Muslim bank balance and property value is paid (zakat).

5. A pilgrimage to Mecca at least once in a lifetime (haj).

The local mosque is built and maintained by the local community of Muslims. It is a place for prayer, a free evening meal after evening prayer session, and free overnight accommodations for Muslim travelers. The Imam is a religious leader and counselor in the Muslim community. He lives at the mosque and is responsible for social, educational, economic, health, and religious welfare.

The Islamic calendar is based on lunar months. A lunar month can be 29 or 30 days long, and the year is 355 days long. Because of this, a Muslim's age will be calculated differently. Eid Day is a festival celebrated at the end of Ramadan. Children are expected to begin fasting at age twelve for a few days, and the number of days increases as they become older.

Adultery and gambling are forbidden. Consumption of alcohol, tobacco, pork, and lard are also taboo. Chicken and other meat must be prepared in a specific manner. Other Islamic taboos include owning statues, images, pictures, photographs, jazz, dogs, and crosses. Sex education, postmortem examinations, and cremation are also forbidden.

Muslim women must wear a veil (purdah) in the presence of males who are not members of the extended family. Muslims also wear thirty-three beads around the neck or wrist to represent the ninety-nine names of God.

Cleanliness is highly valued in Islamic culture. Couples are expected to shower and wash after sexual intercourse. The pig is a symbol of uncleanliness because it lives in a sty. Dogs are also considered unclean. Images are believed to imitate God's creations, so Muslims may refuse even passport pictures.

The preservation of the body after death is important because of the belief in life after death. Muslims venerate graves and value visits to graves and shrines for the dead.

Muslims have a health belief in five therapies which they may use singularly or intermixed. There are scientific medicines, Hakim's remedies (sometimes contaminated with lead), faith healing (largely amulets and charms), religious therapy, and food therapy. Muslims also believe in fate. Muslim women usually have been touched by only one man, their husband, and would prefer a female physician.

Sikhism

At the end of the fifteenth century, Guru Nanak founded Sikhism in Northern India. He rejected the caste system, combined the beliefs of Hindus and Muslims, and believed in a single God. The Sikh believe in both Karma and reincarnation. The worship of idols and representation of God in pictures is forbidden. Guru Nanak had nine masters and followers whose writings were compelled into Sri Guru Grauth Sahib.

There is no specific birth rite, but a newborn is taken to the temple to be named. There is no set age for baptism, which is an important ceremony. However, the individual must be capable of assuming responsibility before the ceremony is performed.

Baptized Sikhs wear turbans and do not cut their hair or shave. All confirmed Sikhs wear five symbols:

—Kesh (uncut hair)

—Kangha (comb)

—Kara (steel bangle, usually worn on the right wrist of both men and women)

—Kacha (pair of white undershorts, symbolic of chastity)

—Kirpan (short sword—8 inches and sheathed).

Baptized men and women do not smoke or use alcohol. They may chew betel, which does contain tobacco, but they do not smoke hooka. Many Sikhs are vegetarians, but this is a matter of choice.

Both social and religious activities are held at the temple. Prayer ceremonies are held daily.

Contraception is discouraged and procreation highly valued. Parental consent is needed for marriage and is usually arranged. Abortion is condoned but is done for sex selection only. Courtship is not allowed.

Sikhs typically have three names: a personal name, a title, and a family name. A woman takes her husband's surname upon marriage. Similar to other Indians, the traditional Sikh greeting is with the palms of the hands pressed together in front of the chest. Women do not shake hands. Direct eye contact is considered rude and disrespectful. Sikh men are not allowed to cut their hair at all. Shaving of infants' heads occurs before the naming ritual and is commonly practiced.

The family, the most important unit in society, is patriarchal. An extended family, it includes brothers, sisters, grandparents, and their families. The life style is collective and interdependent, and earnings are often pooled. Decisions are made by the financially secure male. Sometimes the grandmother is given responsibility for household finances, while the daughter-in-law receives an allowance and manages the household. The mother is responsible for caring for the children. However, health care decisions may be made by senior members of the family, including elderly people, who are respected and have authority. They may also have the responsibility to arrange marriages and help raise grandchildren. As parents age, their sons take care of them. In a majority of cases the parents live with their sons. There is no Social Security or retirement income for the vast majority of Indians. Traditionally they have depended on their sons.

Marriages are arranged, matching status and background, with consultation of horoscopes. In marriage, the woman is given to her husband and his family. Because the man is the breadwinner, the bride's contribution is a dowry. The bride is expected to be a virgin. A girl who even dated is not a suitable marriage prospect; it is believed that "the less you know of others, the more you stick to one." Girls usually marry between the ages of nineteen and twenty-three, on the theory that if they are young, they will adapt more easily. Sex-roles are well defined in the traditional Indian culture, and a wife is traditionally considered her husband's "possession." She must obey him and be submissive, not totally unlike Western culture. At social gatherings, men and women interact and mingle separately. However, the social dignity of the family depends largely on the purity of the daughter before marriage.

Male children are preferred. Traditionally, the extended family and its joint household performed important economic, religious, and social functions. Within the extended family, men still form the framework of continuity. It is believed that a major function of the family is to perpetuate itself through the production of male heirs. When a daughter marries she is considered part of her husband's family and her responsibilities shift to his household. There is also the liability of the expense involved in providing a dowry for a daughter's marriage. The dowry is given in lieu of a share in property, which normally goes to the sons.

Society dictates strict rules and regulations that affect daily life. Independence is discouraged, especially in girls, who are protected, while boys must learn to deal with the outside world. Participation in school activities may be denied or severely restricted because of familial obligations or responsibilities. Sex education is not taught in schools.

The caste system in India has been in existence since ancient times. There are thousands of castes and, though there is consensus as to lower and upper ends of the scale, the intermediate steps vary from village to village. Even in North America, intercaste marriages are unusual. Segmentation also extends to a social class system: professional, intermediate, skilled, semi-skilled, and unskilled. An individual can change social class, but not caste. Information about an individual's caste may or may not be obtained from their name. The first name is the given name, and the middle name is usually the father's name or family name; however, this practice varies from region to region. This may be all the information a provider can obtain when taking a family history.

Divorce and separation are rare, because they would stigmatize the entire family. Parents and respected religious leaders will try to help resolve differences. It is more acceptable for a man to initiate divorce. Traditionally, widows do not remarry. *Suttee* (Sati), the immolation of a Hindu widow on her husband's funeral pyre, has been outlawed, but many other societal behaviors and obligations are intertwined with religion.

BELIEFS ABOUT HEALTH

Ayurvedic medicine is the ancient Indian medical system. Imbalance in the body humors (bile, urine, and phlegm) results in illness. *Ayur* means "life" or "life span," and *Veda* means "knowledge" or "science"; therefore, it is translated to mean "science of life." It is a science that emphasizes homeostasis. The physiological principles are called *doshas:* Vata, Pitta, Kapha.

Dosha	Imbalance	Conditions
Vata	Motion and flow	Nervous system problems, chronic pain, cardiac arrhythmia, anxiety, constipation, insomnia
Pitta	Directs all metabolic activities	Peptic ulcers, hypertension, allergic reactions, bowel disease
Kapha	Structure and cohesion	Disease of respiratory system, sinusitis, diabetes, obesity, tumors

The emphasis of treatment is to restore balance. Every patient receives recommendations for therapy for the mind and body. Therapy is based on imbalance in doshas rather than disease type.

There are various causes and sources of imbalance, and diet is a common etiology. According to Ayurvedic medicine, excesses such as immorality, alcohol, and sex can also lead to sickness. The "evil eye," or possession by a demon, it holds, may cause mental illness.

Treatments vary, but balance must be regained. Foods are considered "hot" and "cold" and must be eaten appropriately. Other cures consist of bathing (or its avoidance), massage, and herbal teas. For high levels of stress, a priest or exorcist performs ritualistic chants in the individual's home. The ceremony may end with a protective thread to be worn by the individual.

In rural areas, the barber may be the specialist in bone-setting or treating snake bites. Astrologers and palm readers may be consulted. Trained Ayurvedic physicians, who attend Ayurvedic college and hold diplomas to practice medicine employ Western biomedical techniques and instruments, such as stethoscopes and pulse-taking. Individuals also use home remedies and, to keep cost to a minimum, do not go to the physician until the illness is severe.

Although Western medicine is employed, many Asian Indians believe Ayurvedic treatment is more natural and has fewer side effects. There are also "infectionists," who supply Western-type drugs. For approximately every thirty-six hundred people, there is one Western-type physician, and his or her fees may be expensive for the average family. Midwives deliver babies at home, as well as provide the prenatal and postnatal care. Hospitals are for serious illnesses.

Medical decisions are made by the family. The choice of whether to visit the physician may rest with the head of the household. Great trust is put in physicians of both traditional and Western training. It is expected that the physician will have all the answers and make the decisions. Social distance between the doctor and patient may be very great, so the interaction is formal. The doctor's dress should also be formal. Hospital clothing presents a problem, since the patient hesitates to wear clothing used by others, even if washed and sterilized. There are superstitions attaching harmful effects to used clothing on newborn infants. Newborns are protected from exposure to strangers because of concerns that infection could lead to mortality.

Surgery is accepted only after a detailed explanation, and an astrologer may be consulted to decide the day. Organ transplants and blood transfusions are not forbidden by any religious beliefs. The sacred thread worn by high-caste Hindus should not be cut without the family's permission. Rectal exams are offensive. In certain sects, enemas are taboo, but elsewhere they are utilized.

Death is considered a part of the life cycle. Each religious community has its own specific practices and rituals. Fatalism is a strong belief; death comes when it is time for the person to die. Muslims believe it is determined by Allah, while Hindus and Sikhs believe it is determined by one's Karma. Death is preferable at home surrounded by family. Grief is open and very vocal. Not to demonstrate grief in that manner would subject one to criticism.

Pregnancy is considered a normal, healthy state. Therefore, a physician is not consulted. Life continues as usual: work in the fields, sex, and the same diet. However, "hot" foods are avoided in the first trimester, because of the belief that they might cause miscarriage and premature birth. The pregnant woman, particularly when pregnant for the first time, is well taken care of and greatly pampered. This indicates that she is fertile and the family will continue in the next generation.

IMPLICATIONS FOR GENETIC SERVICES

At the beginning of the session, greetings should be formal, and it may be best to address the elders and males first. Then the genetic counselor should try to assess the degree of acculturation of the family and their expectations from the session. The Asian Indian has respect for the physician and expects a diagnosis and treatment. It would be helpful to explain how the genetic counseling session differs from other medical encounters. Indirect counseling may not be well understood.

Decision-making may be done by the family, and consideration should be given to this if the patient needs to have a second appointment for tests or for other reasons. Diagnostic tests should be explained thoroughly. Carrier testing is not done in India and may mean stigmatization if an individual is found to carry an altered gene. This is especially a consideration whenever arranged marriages are undertaken. If it is perceived that a wife is "defective," the husband may divorce her or make a request for a second marriage. This is an important and serious concern when discussing X-linked recessive disorders and autosomal dominant disorders. Moreover, in the discussion of the latter, providers must understand that both people are carriers and should minimize blame, feelings of guilt, and low self-esteem.

Family information can present challenges. For many first-generation immigrants, age may not be precise because birth records were not kept until recently. Age is calculated by association with an important event or celebration. Men and women may disclose different information about the family. Women have the care of the children and may address such matters, while men may discuss other issues. Again, privacy and confidentiality should be assured. Marriages between cousins are not unusual, and the counselor should be careful not to be judgmental. While many individuals may expect a good physician to gather a complete history, others may resent or regard as irrelevant the in-depth history-taking in genetics.

Amniocentesis and ultrasound are being used in India for sex selection, since male children are preferred, especially as the first born. This practice could alter the male to female population ratio in some areas. If there is a prohibition policy preventing sex selection, this should be explained and disclosed to the patient.

Artificial insemination by donor is probably a new concept to many. It should be presented as an option offered in Western culture and not a recommendation. GIFT and in vitro fertilization may be acceptable. Adoption is well accepted.

Autopsies may be declined by Hindus and Sikhs, while Muslims may consent only if legally necessary. The Sikhs, because of religious beliefs, most likely will participate in organ donation.

Other practices and cultural issues that may arise in the counseling session include: children with disabilities, who are taken care of by the family; institutional commitment is not common. Photographs of affected children may not be permitted by Sikhs or Muslims. Although there are many "superstitions," taboo numbers do not seem to be a problem. Informed consent as a part of the Western medical system may not be well understood.

Nonverbal communication is important. Direct eye contact is considered disrespectful. Women especially are not touched, except by their husbands. (It would be less traumatic to assign a female geneticist if a physical exam is needed.) Grief is displayed and expected, but silence or blushing may occur in response to embarrassing situations.

Avoidance of idioms and jargon is important in the discussion. Visual aids of chromosomes, etc., may be helpful. Many medical expressions are not understood by the average American. Many expressions are learned early in life and an individual, no matter how facile in English, may not understand expressions such as a "period," in reference to a woman's menstrual cycle.

The incidence of divorce and separation is exceedingly low. Nonpaternity rarely occurs in traditional families. Alcoholism is extremely low, especially among women, so concomitantly would be the incidence of fetal alcohol syndrome. In fact, some Muslims may not want to be in the waiting room with others who may use alcohol. These families may wish to be the last appointment of the day to minimize such contact.

CONCLUSION

Asian Indians do not constitute a cohesive community in most parts of the United States, in contrast to Canada. Many are well educated and have professional jobs, but do not have the social support and structure of their religion. India is not a homogeneous society; diversity is the rule. New immigrants face economic stresses and strains, which may have resulted from discrimination. Many individuals may be hesitant or fear the counseling session. This fear can be minimized by a polite and patient counselor, who needs to listen carefully as well as be clear in explanations. Interpreters should be picked who are culturally appropriate. When in doubt, ask. The English that many East Indians speak is the queen's English, and idioms and jargon are different and can create confusion.

SUMMARY

—Address males and elders first; keep greetings formal.

—Explain how genetic counseling differs from other health care encounters and the importance of the in-depth family history.

—For first-generation immigrants, age may not precisely be known, because birth records are a recent innovation.

—Explain diagnostic tests thoroughly. Carrier testing can lead to discrimination and difficulty if marriages are arranged.

—Allow for two clinic visits if possible; decision-making may be done by all family members and tests may not be accomplished until the next visit.

—Explain the clinic or facility philosophy about sex selection if it has a bearing on the counseling session.

—Adoption is well accepted.

—Sikhs and Hindus may decline autopsies. Muslims may consent if legally necessary.

—If appropriate, mention being left-handed at the beginning of the session. Some individuals may consider this a sign of bad luck.

—Learn the special holidays or celebrations. Do not schedule clinic visits on these days (i.e., Husband's Day, Brother's Day).

—In traditional Sikh families, women do not shake hands. Learn the traditional greeting of palms of hands pressed together in the front of the chest.

—Explain informed consent.

—Visual aids may be helpful.

—Avoid idioms and jargon. Asians Indians speak English well; however, it is the queen's English and its nuances and language are different.

—In traditional families, nonpaternity rarely occurs.

—Surgical procedures are not readily accepted and detailed information should be provided.

—Women are usually touched only by their husbands. Be mindful of this when greeting, offering consolation, performing a physical examination, and other types of contact.

—Fatalism may be a strong belief and individuals may not be as stressed about the results of tests that Westerners consider bad news.

REFERENCES

Assamand, S., et al. 1990. *The South Asians in Cross-Cultural Caring: A Handbook for Health Professionals in Western Canada.* Vancouver: University of British Columbia Press.

Balodhi, J. P. 1992. Indian mythological views on suicide. *Nimhans Journal* 10:101–5.

Chaduri, R. 1992. Self-determination: Lessons to be learnt from social work practice in India: A comment. *British Journal of Social Work* 22:187–91.

Cheng, L. R. 1990. Asian-American cultural perspectives on birth defects: Focus on cleft palate. *Cleft Palate Journal* 27:294–300.

Florsheim, P. 1990. Cross-cultural views on self in the treatment of mental illness: Disentangling the curative aspects of myth from the mythic aspects of cure. *Psychiatry* 53:304–15.

Geissler, E. M. 1993. *Pocket Guide to Cultural Assessment.* St. Louis: Mosby.

Johnson, A. M., and Nadirhaw, Z. 1993. Good practice in transcultural counseling: An Asian perspective. *British Journal of Guidance Counselling* 21:20–29.

Larson, J. H., and Medora, N. 1992. Privacy preferences: A cross-cultural comparison of American and Asian Indians. *International Journal of Sociology of the Family* 22:55–66.

Murthy, R. S., Subramanian, K. V., and Chatterji, S. 1990. Psychiatric research in India: Annual review, 1988. *Nimhans Journal* 8:13–21.

Naveed, M., Phadke, S. R., Sharma, A., and Agarwal, S. S. 1992. Sociocultural problems in genetic counseling. *Journal of Medical Genetics* 29:140.

Pinto, A., Folkers, E., and Sines, J. D. 1991. Dimensions of behavior and home environment in school-age children: India and United States. *Journal of Cross-Cultural Psychiatry* 22:491–508.

Qureshi, B. 1989. *Transcultural Medicine: Principles and Practice.* London: Kluwer Academic Publishers.

Ramakrishna, J., and Weiss, M. G. 1992. Health, illness, and immigration: East Indians in the United States. *Western Journal of Medicine* 157:265–70.

Sharma, H. M., Triguna, B. D., and Chopra, D. 1991. Maharishi Ayur-Veda: Modern insights into ancient medicine. *Journal of the American Medical Association* 265:2633–34.

Ullrich, H. E. 1992. Menstrual taboos among Havik Brahmin women: A study of ritual change. *Sex Roles* 26:19–40.

10

Christian Culture in North America

David C. Koehn, M.Sc., and
Rose Anne Pillay, B.Sc., B.Ed.

A Christian is defined as "one who believes Jesus is the Christ and Son of God and the way to salvation is through Him" (Bentley, 1983). Though this definition is relatively straightforward, in actual fact, two thousand years of history have brought about tremendous diversity among Christian believers. Christianity has grown from an obscure Jewish cult into one of the world's most widespread and largest religions. There are currently more than one billion Christians worldwide (Bentley, 1983) and the number continues to increase.

HISTORY

The Christian movement began shortly after the death and resurrection of Jesus Christ, when, according to Christian belief, the Holy Spirit empowered Jesus's disciples with the mission to spread the news of Christ to the world. Paul, an early church leader who became a follower after Christ's death, was instrumental in transforming the faith from one held initially by Jews to one that was universally recognized. His letters gave advice on moral issues to developing Christian communities and helped form Christian doctrine. Christianity broke conventional barriers of race and status, and an equality of mutual affection predominated within the community of believers.

The early efforts of Christians to evangelize met with much hostility and persecution, and yet the fledgling movement flourished. Persecution has often been a part of church history, and the doctrine that suffering for one's faith is an ideal that has become entrenched. James 1:2 states, "Consider it all joy, my brethren, when you encounter various trials, knowing that the testing of your faith produces endurance" (New American Standard Version). This ideal may, in combination with other issues to be discussed, cause a couple to decide to continue with an abnormal pregnancy. It also may allow a couple to endure the significant burden of a severely handicapped child with acceptance and perseverance.

In A.D. 313, Christianity became a legally recognized religion within the Roman Empire (Smith, 1958) due to a sympathetic emperor, Constantine. He initiated the council of Nicea in 325 as the first formal attempt to standardize the already diverse forms of Christianity and its doctrines. Before the century was out (380), Christianity had become the official religion of the Roman Empire. It continued, for the most part, as a united organization until 1054 (Smith, 1958).

DENOMINATIONS

The Christian Church is divided into three major branches: Roman Catholicism, Eastern Orthodoxy, and Protestantism (Smith, 1958). Roman Catholicism is centered in the Vatican in Rome and spreads from there, being dominant through Central and Southern Europe, Ireland, and South America. Eastern Orthodoxy has its major influence in Greece, the Slavic countries, and Russia. Protestantism dominates Northern Europe, England, Scotland, and North America. From these three major branches have evolved well over a thousand groups and subgroups known as denominations, particularly in relation to Protestantism (Bentley, 1983). Each denomination or group has a slightly different concept of what it means to be a Christian in terms of principles and practices and maintains a distinct flavor of its own based on linguistic, cultural, or historic roots.

Roman Catholicism

Roman Catholicism, the largest unified organization, with over six hundred million members (Bentley, 1983), honors Peter as the chosen leader of the disciples of Christ. Peter's successor, the pope, heads a hierarchical organization that manages church affairs down to the smallest parish, and is the final authority on doctrine. There has been a succession of popes since Peter. In the hierarchy of the church under the pope are cardinals, archbishops, bishops, and priests.

The Roman Catholic Church sees itself as the ultimate teaching authority on all matters of salvation: how people should live in this world so as to attain eternal life in the next. The church attempts to resolve moral issues for its followers to unify belief. Catholic individuals may wish to enlist the aid of a priest in their decision-making. However, it should be noted that the priest may not be comfortable dealing with prenatal decision-making, where the church's views may contradict the couple's wishes.

The Catholic Church, as well as other Christian denominations, believes in the concept of "original sin"; every human is born sinful. Mankind can never be perfect of its own accord. The key to salvation is through seven sacraments. St. Augustine called such rites "a visible form of an invisible grace." They were defined at the second council of Lyons in 1274 (Whalen, 1971). As described by Smith (1958, p. 296),

> The sacraments provide the spiritual counterpart to man's natural existence. As birth brings a child into the natural world, *baptism* draws him into the supernatural order or existence. When he reaches the age of reason and needs to be strengthened for mature and responsible action, he is *confirmed*. Usually there comes a solemn moment when he is joined to a human companion in *holy matrimony*, or dedicates his life entirely to God and his work in *holy orders*. At the end of his life, *extreme unction* (last rites) closes his eyes to earth and prepares his soul for its last passage.

Issues surrounding the sacraments of baptism and death will be discussed later. Confirmation and dedication of one's life to God's service are relatively straightforward. There are some issues relating to the sacrament of marriage that should be addressed. Marriage within the Catholic Church is the ideal, but marriage outside of the church is not prohibited. Polygamy is banned. Divorce is prohibited; marriage is sacred and until death. Under special circumstances, annulments are granted by the Vatican. The stipulation is that all children should be brought up in the Catholic Church.

Sexual intercourse deepens the sacramental commitment and allows for procreation. Adultery is not condoned by the church, so one may be less likely to find cases of nonpaternity with DNA testing among those who adhere strictly to the church's teaching. The church advocates natural family planning (rhythm, monitoring body temperature) as a means by which couples can regulate the timing and number of births. The use of other forms of contraception is considered a sin. Selection for a sex or a particular trait is considered morally illicit (DeMarco, 1987). The church discourages consanguineous marriages, stemming perhaps from concerns relating to rare disorders arising from such unions. However, consanguineous couples can receive a special dispensation from a Vatican committee if they wish to marry. In vitro fertilization, artificial insemination by a donor, sperm banks, surrogate motherhood, and test tube babies are not condoned by the church because they affect the sacrament of holy matrimony.

Catholics need to repeat two sacraments on an ongoing basis (Smith, 1958). Confession, or reconciliation, reestablishes human community and divine fellowship when a person has erred. The church teaches that if a person confesses sin to God in the presence of a priest and truly repents, he or she will be forgiven. The second and central sacrament of the Roman Catholic Church is the Mass. Mass is a reenactment of Christ's Last Supper and is used to elevate the spirit individually as well as communally. The Catholic view of the Mass or communion differs from those of other Christian denominations because Catholics believe that the elements (bread and wine) are miraculously transformed into the actual body and blood of Christ and hence Mass is not merely a commemoration or remembrance but an act of spiritual nourishment. For Catholic and Eastern Orthodox patients, one must be sensitive to the importance of these sacraments and uphold them in situations deemed necessary, such as baptism or Communion.

One further belief specific to the Roman Catholic Church is the view of intercessors. Catholics believe that the Virgin Mary (Christ's mother) and other saints can intercede for the faithful and can act in the communication process between God and mankind in certain circumstances. Prayer can often provide guidance in difficult situations.

In recent times, positions have expanded on birth control, divorce, women's position in the church, and other issues. Consequently, the practices of many Catholics worldwide vary greatly.

Eastern Orthodoxy

The Eastern Schism was the result of almost two hundred years of controversy between Rome and Constantinople. It erupted over complex geographic, linguistic, cultural, political, and religious roots. In 1054, the Eastern Orthodox church was formalized under the leadership of the Patriarch of Constantinople. The Eastern Orthodox Church today has sixteen major divisions, including the Greek Orthodox, the Russian Orthodox, and the Ukrainian Orthodox. There are about one hundred million followers worldwide (Bentley, 1983).

Each of the churches in Eastern Orthodoxy is self-governing, continuing the patriarchates of early Christianity. The sixteen autonomous branches, however, are in full communion with one another, and their members see themselves as belonging to the Eastern Church. There is a very strong corporate feeling within the Eastern Church. Each Christian is working out salvation with the rest of the church, not individually, to save his or her own soul (Smith, 1958).

In contrast to the hierarchical nature of the Roman Catholic Church, the Eastern Orthodox Church rests more of its decisions with the laity. The members of each congregation elect their own clergy. Without this election, the bishop cannot appoint leadership. The line that separates clergy from laity, beyond the administration of sacraments, is thin. Eastern Orthodoxy maintains that the Holy Spirit's truth is diffused throughout the collective church, and encourages the mystical tradition in its adherents. The Patriarch of Constantinople is merely "the first among equals" and the laity is known as "the royal priesthood" (Smith, 1958). Hence, the Eastern Church rejects the pope as head of the Christian Church.

In many ways, however, the Eastern Orthodox Church stands close to the Roman Catholic Church. It honors the seven sacraments and interprets them similarly to the Catholic Church (Smith, 1958). There are surface differences in that the Eastern Church uses unleavened bread in the Holy Communion and rejects transubstantiation (Bentley, 1983). The Catholic Church frequently reserves the cup, while the Eastern Church offers it along with the bread. Priests can marry and do not take a vow of celibacy in the Eastern Church (Bentley, 1983).

The Eastern Orthodox Church, like the Roman Catholic Church, sees itself as an authority on spiritual issues but differs, first, in the extent to which unanimity is required. Only issues mentioned in Scripture can qualify (Smith, 1958). The church can interpret doctrines but it cannot initiate them. In practice, it has interpreted on only seven occasions, embodied in its creeds. The last Ecumenical Council was in A.D. 78 (Smith, 1958), hence tradition is often seen as the guide of the church. Issues such as purgatory, indulgences, immaculate conception, or the bodily assumption of Mary were all defined by the Roman Catholic Church after the Schism and are not part of the Eastern Orthodox tradition. The Eastern Church leaves many more issues open to individual judgment, though tradition dictates strongly. Eastern Orthodox priests do not usually serve as clergy in North American hospitals. Second, the Eastern Orthodox Church differs in the way decisions on issues are reached. The Catholic Church sees the ultimate authority on all decisions to be the pope, whereas the Eastern Church believes more in a consensus of Christians focused through ecclesiastical councils. A collective judgment establishes God's truth.

Protestantism

The causes that led to the Protestant Reformation and a further break from the Roman Catholic tradition are as complex as those that resulted in the Great Schism. Political economy, nationalism, individualism, and a rising concern over the abuses of the church all played a role. Primarily, however, the central cause was a difference in religious perspective. Protestants maintain that the Bible is the final authority on all issues and that salvation is a gift of God, available to all who believe and not obtained through the dictates of the church. Faith in Christ is central to this belief. Protestant Christianity contains many denominations within its boundaries and can be defined much more as a movement than as a single unified church (Smith, 1958).

The Protestant movement began in the sixteenth century and has increased in its diversity with time. Today, an Anglican church as well as a Southern Pentecostal church would be considered Protestant, though they vary greatly in religious practice.

The Protestant Church is rooted in the history of the Reform movement in Europe. Some reformers, such as Martin Luther, felt it was adequate to remodel the existing Roman Catholic Church, with changes that were more in tune with the doctrine and practices of Scriptures. Luther rejected Rome and emphasized "justification by faith alone" while maintaining a formal liturgy and a state church (Hillerbrand, 1971). Others, like the Calvinists or Reformed church, following the teachings of John Calvin, sought to change the existing church completely, to make it more like what they saw the New Testament church to be in the Scriptures. They combined this with a doctrine of predestination. English developments (Anglican) were unique in combining advanced doctrine with a fairly conservative form of church government, with the monarch of England as its head (Walls, 1985). More radical streams of Protestantism held that if faith was a personal trust in God, then the church could consists of only those who truly believed, and did not consist of the entire population of the state.

These closely knit fellowships of families began to be known as Anabaptists because of their rejection of the practice of infant baptism. Modern-day equivalents of the Anabaptists are the Baptists, Congregationalists, Mennonites, and Quakers (Walls, 1985). Some of these small, radical Protestant groups, such as the Hutterites or Amish, due to their separate life style and limited outbreeding, have been of importance to the delineation of a variety of genetic disorders (see chapter 11).

It would be difficult to describe in detail the differences between the thousand different denominations of Protestant churches today, but suffice it to say that many started from these early roots, and flourished under the direction of charismatic leaders. The majority are based on a particular group's emphasis or interpretation of Scripture. For example, Pentecostal churches, most of whose original members were once Baptists or Methodists but which now incorporate many different revivalist groups, have a particular emphasis on the work of the Holy Spirit, specifically manifesting itself in divine healing and speaking in tongues (Hillerbrand, 1971). Other large Protestant denominations not previously mentioned are Adventist, Christian Church (Disciples of Christ), Church of Christ, Methodist, Presbyterian, Episcopal, and United Church.

In dealing with couples or individuals from a Protestant background, it would be wise to ask about their particular belief system regarding a particular issue and not to assume anything. Individualism, after all, is a hallmark of the Protestants.

Nonmainstream Groups

Through the centuries, many groups have separated themselves from mainstream Christian thought. Though they are often grouped as Protestant because they are not of the Roman Catholic tradition, we treat them separately here because of the doctrinal differences in their teachings from mainstream Christianity, specifically relating to Jesus Christ and the Trinity.

The Church of Jesus Christ of Latter Day Saints (Mormons) was established in 1830 in New York under the leadership of Joseph Smith. This church is based on the continued revelation of God to mankind, and specifically the Book of Mormon, which was the revelation given to Joseph Smith. The early Mormons were persecuted for their beliefs, which led them to head west to Salt Lake City, Utah, where they finally settled and set up a church state. There are approximately five million Mormon followers today (Bentley, 1983). Revelation continues through the president of the church. Unique to Mormon beliefs is baptism for the dead and sealing in marriage for eternity (Hillerbrand, 1971). Polygamy, though an original belief of the church, has been prohibited since 1890. Contrary to public opinion, Mormons do not have arranged marriages. Through extensive genealogies, the Mormons in Utah have made an important contribution to the delineation of recessive genetic diseases and population inbreeding. Recessive diseases in this group, as in all isolates, are related to a small gene pool and not conscious consanguinity.

The Church of Christ, Scientist, was founded in 1879 by Mary Baker Eddy on the basis of a theological distinction between the Divine Mind (God, life, truth) and the mortal mind (sin, disease, error). Christian Scientists reject medical treatment. "Practitioners" heal by prayer and divine law (Hillerbrand, 1971).

Jehovah's Witnesses was established in 1884 by Charles Taze Russell. Instead of believing that Christ's second coming is imminent, they believe that his second presence took place in 1914 and he has ruled, invisibly from heaven, since that time. Jehovah's Witnesses, like Mormons, are persistent in spreading their beliefs because of their view that only a select group will actually gain access to heaven. They refuse to participate in worldly politics or the military. They also refuse to allow their children to have blood transfusions, based on an Old Testament injunction against eating blood (Genesis 9:3,4; Bentley, 1983). This latter refusal can make it necessary for a hospital to apply to a court to transfuse blood into a child who needs surgery to correct a congenital anomaly, and one needs to be prepared for this in the practice of medical genetics. Synthetic alternatives to blood transfusion, such as dextrin, fluosol (Bentley, 1983), and erythropoietin, are currently being developed and utilized.

BELIEFS

God

Christians worship the God of Israel referenced in Jewish scriptures. God is seen as beneficent, all-powerful, all-knowing, universal, and a creator and guide of the people. God is part of a Trinity (one God in three distinct persons) composed of God, Jesus Christ (God's son), and the Holy Spirit. God transcends as well as acts in history. The earliest Christians, being Jewish, knew this deity from the history of their nation and their Scriptures. Greek Christians were able to meld the God of the Bible with the God of philosophical tradition, who was known to be the Ultimate

Good or Unknown God. Ultimately, Christians were able to see themselves as continuous with the nation of Israel, a people set apart by God, and to see the biblical history of Israel as part of their own (Walls, 1985).

The diagnosis of an abnormality or disability in a child sometimes shakes a Christian's belief in a beneficent God. A couple may believe that God is somehow no longer acting on their behalf or else is affecting their lives in this way as a form of judgment for sins they committed or to test their faith. Though the God of the Old Testament did act in judgment, the New Testament shows God's overall compassion. To reduce patients' guilt and blame, it is important for health professionals to emphasize that the birth of a child with congenital anomalies is not personally directed.

Jesus Christ and the Holy Spirit

The term *Christian* was first used around A.D. 35–40 in Antioch in Syria to describe a group of people who demonstrated attachment to "Christos" (Walls, 1985; Acts 2:26). This was a Greek translation of the Hebrew word *Messiah,* used by Jews to designate their expected national savior. This new movement, originating from Jewish sources, identified the Messiah with the recent Jesus of Nazareth. Allegiance to Christ and his teachings and life style has remained crucial to every Christian denomination.

To understand Christianity, one must have a knowledge of the person of Christ. He was born in Israel during the time of Herod the Great. He was a Jew by birth, yet it is believed that his heritage was both human and divine (divine incarnation). He began his ministry on earth at the age of thirty, teaching about the divine plan of salvation. The culmination of this plan was his death by crucifixion and resurrection. The Holy Spirit as an intangible presence was left as a comforter and guide to believers, especially with regard to decision-making on issues of morality.

Certain features are common to the various Christian perceptions of the significance of Jesus (Walls, 1985). First, Jesus Christ has to be interpreted in the light of the fact that Christians worship the God of Israel. This does not compromise previous monotheistic thought, since Jesus and God are thought to be one. God is present and active in the world, particularly through Jesus Christ and / or the Holy Spirit.

Second, Jesus provides the moral yardstick for the believer. Jesus is the moral absolute in all forms of Christianity. When making decisions in a difficult ethical situation, Christians often ask, "What would Christ have done?" This questions can guide some couples in their decision-making process when they face the difficult choices that are part of some medical genetic situations. Would termination of a fetus with Down syndrome be an option?

Third, the ultimate significance of Jesus is bound up in his death and its outcome. Jesus's death was on behalf of others. It was associated with God's forgiveness of humanity, and the resurrection of Christ was associated with God's triumph over death. There has followed from it the promise of the eventual resurrection of the human race as well as the accessibility of God's living presence. The underlying conviction is that Jesus will bring world history to a climax and establish a new kingdom.

Finally, Jesus Christ's words, his actions, and the person he was have had an impact far beyond his time. All the words Jesus spoke in the New Testament can be said in two hours (Smith, 1958), yet they are the most repeated words in the world. His messages, parables, and beatitudes focus on two issues: God's overwhelming love for humanity, and the need for people to receive this love and let it flow outward again toward their neighbors (Smith, 1958). The Christian emphasis on love for all persons will affect a Christian couple's prenatal decision-making, discussed in more detail later. Also from this underlying principle will come a greater acceptance of a child with a genetic condition or disability: "Our disabled brothers and sisters are prophets in our midst giving lie to what others have termed the 'cult of perfection'" (Bevilacqua, 1993). Similarly, based on this principle, adoption is an accepted practice throughout every church denomination and encompasses children with special needs. Since Christians believe that God created all things and loves all things, they view all life as precious and sacred.

Sin

Christianity teaches that humans were originally made in the image of God and were given the freedom to choose between good and evil. However, the first humans, Adam and Eve, disobeyed God, and the result of that disobedience or sin was separation from God and awareness of guilt for the entire human race (Little, 1985). God provided a redemptive plan to reestablish a relationship with humankind through the sacrifice of his son, Jesus Christ, to pay the ultimate penalty for all sin, which is death. Protestants obtain redemption through confession of sin and belief in the forgiveness of Christ. Members of the Eastern Orthodox and Roman Catholic churches seek redemption through these same principles combined with observance of the sacraments.

The Roman Catholic Church has a well-developed doctrine surrounding the concept of sin. Original sin, incurred through Adam and Eve and affecting all mankind, can be expiated by baptism at birth. Venial sin, encompassing sins that are not willfully done but are part of everyday life (e.g., a white lie), can be cleansed through penance or in purgatory. Mortal sins, which are willful transgressions, condemn one to hell but can be forgiven. Mortal sins include a spectrum ranging from missing Mass to murder and include contraception, in vitro fertilization, artificial insemination by a donor, surrogate motherhood, and abortion. In contrast, most Protestants would not consider contraception or assisted reproduction to be a sin and would be more likely to weigh each issue on a case-by-case basis.

The concepts of sin and guilt are often critical to couples who decide to terminate a pregnancy for genetic concerns and are difficult to overcome. One must be sensitive in such a situation. It may be helpful to emphasize that God is still there and will provide forgiveness. A couple may need to discuss this issue with their clergy. Roman Catholics, due to their strong focus on sin, may have greater difficulty in accepting this forgiveness, as their decision was a willful choice in direct contradiction with the moral guidelines of the church.

The Bible

The Bible, believed by Christians to be inspired by God and comprising the Old and New Testaments, is the source of Christian doctrine and regulates church life. Christians have adopted the Jewish scriptures as their own in the form of the Old Testament (Walls, 1985). Many passages are felt to relate to Christ and reflect a process of divine revelation of which he was the climax. The New Testament contains writings about the life of Christ as well as the doctrines of the early church.

Public reading of the Bible has always been a feature of Christian worship, although private reading was reinstituted following the Protestant Reformation. Protestants strongly emphasize personal interpretation or illumination of biblical passages, while Roman Catholics and Eastern Orthodox rely more heavily on the church authority regarding interpretation. Differences in interpretation and the accessibility to translation have much to do with the immense cultural adaptations that have been a hallmark of Christianity.

Many Christians take comfort in difficult situations or aid their decision-making by referring to passages in the Bible. One such passage is Psalms 23:4, which states, "Even though I walk through the valley of the shadow of death, I fear no evil; for Thou art with me; Thy rod and Thy staff, they comfort me" (New American Standard Version).

Community / People of God

Christians feel a degree of continuity with the people of Israel and carry over Israel's sense of being a people of God. This results in a doctrine of the church transcending time, space, and race. Different groups interpret in different ways how the church's corporate body is identified and expressed in time and locality.

The church community can provide a variety of resources, ranging from guidance and counseling to support and self-help initiatives. It is a place to which believers turn in times of difficulty. The ethical decisions or situations that are often a part of medical genetic practice may motivate this search. When a child dies or a miscarriage occurs, the couple has access to a supportive network. If an individual has physical or mental disabilities, the church may help foster that person's social and spiritual development in a supportive environment (e.g., L'arch community, a Roman Catholic hospice / group home for the mentally or physically challenged). Practical support for families within a church may involve food, clothing, or respite care. Many churches are affiliated with group homes or societies that reach out to help families in need.

Turning to the church, however, can cause difficulty if the church's views conflict with an individual's personal choices. An unaccepting or unforgiving attitude on the part of some members of the church community can make a difficult situation worse or increase the complexity of the decision-making in processing prenatal issues.

Death

In Christianity, a person's earthly existence is finite. After death, the person's soul is without a body and enters the afterlife. A person dies either as one who has been redeemed or as one who is under judgment (Little, 1985). This means the soul enters either paradise (heaven) or a state of torment (hell). It is the desire of every Christian to be found righteous and go to heaven upon dying. Christ's own resurrection seals this hope, they believe, and the Second Coming of Christ will initiate a final Day of Judgment by God.

The Roman Catholic Church has two further residences of the soul in the afterlife: a state of purgatory, where a soul may be purged of sin before reaching heaven; and a possible state of happiness without God, which is reserved for the unborn and unbaptized as well as the patriarchs who died before the coming of Christ.

The idea that the soul's existence is separate from that of the earthly body allows for the donation of one's body or organs to medical science if one so chooses. In addition, this idea allows for autopsies that aid in diagnosis. However, the Catholic Church feels strongly that an autopsy is necessary only if the cause of death has not been determined. This proviso also applies to corpses of human embryos and fetuses due to therapeutic or social termination or miscarriage and is based on a principle of respect for the remains. Likewise, experimentation on or mutilation of human fetuses is considered morally illicit (DeMarco, 1987).

With regard to funeral rituals, most Christians are embalmed and buried. For some, entombment or cremation is also an option. Funeral services are a remembrance of an individual's life by friends and family. Often specific religious rites, such as the celebration of Mass at a Catholic funeral, need to be observed. Funerals, though sad events because of the grief surrounding the loss of a loved one, are infused with an element of joy due to the hope of an afterlife. This provides comfort to the bereaved.

PRACTICES

The range of Christian practice is as immense as the range of Christian doctrine and is equally impossible to summarize. The syncretistic nature of Christianity means that many Christian elements appear as part of normal social life. Many practices found in other religions also occur in Christianity, but only in certain denominational groups. The Scriptures refer explicitly to many fundamental practices. Beyond this, however, it may be difficult to identify commonality.

Prayer

Prayer is a means of communication with God and can be performed either publicly or privately. It was taught by Jesus (e.g., the Lord's Prayer) and exemplified in the letters of Paul. It is held to be an obligation as well as a privilege through which access can be gained to the transcendent world. Christian prayer is typically addressed to God through the mediation of Jesus Christ, and its motivation and effect are associated with the action of the Holy Spirit.

Christian individuals often use prayer in difficult situations in an attempt to obtain guidance or in supplication. Prayer is crucial in making all life choices. James 5:13–14 states, "Is anyone among you suffering? Let him pray. Is anyone cheerful? Let him sing praises. Is anyone among you sick? Let him call for the elders of the church, and let them pray over him, anointing him with oil in the name of the Lord" (New American Standard Version).

A Christian couple faced with the decision of terminating life-support systems for an infant with severe congenital anomalies may wish to take time to pray about this issue and should be encouraged to do so. Prayer can also be used in a church community setting as a means of corporate support for a couple or individual who are not coping well in a given life situation. Prayer in the public forum increases corporate sensitivity and support.

Days of Observance

Jewish law requires that the seventh day be kept holy or separate from the other days of the week (Walls, 1985). Most Christian groups set apart Sunday, considered the first day of the week and associated with the day of the resurrection of Christ, as a day of worship and a remittance of normal practices. One notable exception is Seventh Day Adventists, who meet on Saturdays.

There are other holy days associated with special services practiced throughout Christendom. Most Christian denominations celebrate Easter (commemorating the resurrection of Christ), Christmas (commemorating the birth of Christ), and Pentecost (celebrating the unleashing of the Holy Spirit on earth). Orthodox, Roman Catholic, and Anglican churches adhere to a structured church year, celebrating these as well as other events associated with Christ, salvation, biblical themes, events, or particular saints (Walls, 1985).

In scheduling appointments for known Christians, one should avoid specific holy days or days of observance if at all possible. One should also be aware that at certain festive times of the year, such as Christmas, it is particularly difficult to deliver news of an abnormal result to a couple. Increased sensitivity is required, as it is often more difficult for the couple or individual to cope with such information, as this holiday is associated with family traditions and high expectations.

Baptism

Baptism, a means of blessing or dedicating a person to God, involving sprinkling or immersion with water, was a rite that was used in Judaism to symbolize the cleansing of a Gentile convert to Judaism. Early Christian followers administered baptism to adult believers as a symbol of a change of heart and entrance into the Christian community. This is the view of many Protestant denominations, especially those with roots in the Anabaptist tradition. Paul associated immersion in water as a symbol of the death, burial, and resurrection of Jesus (Walls, 1985).

It is unclear when the baptism of children began to be practiced. It may have come about at the time Christianity became a state religion, but it is practiced today by Orthodox, Roman Catholic, and some Protestant groups and is considered one of the sacraments. In these denominations it is very important to perform the rite of baptism in vivo on all individuals to wash away the original sin of Adam and Eve, thus allowing for redemption.

Baptism can be performed by any baptized Christian. In cases of late-term pregnancy termination, to ensure that the fetus will enjoy salvation, baptism is recommended for the fetuses that are still alive at birth. Furthermore, if prenatal diagnosis (amniocentesis, chorionic villus sampling, or ultrasound) reveals that the fetus will not be born in the normal manner, then baptism in the womb is recommended. Aborted fetuses that are dead upon removal from the uterus cannot be baptized but may be given a blessing by a priest. Funerals (burials or cremations) are permitted, but the service will be one of memorial as opposed to a Christian funeral rite if the infants are unbaptized (DeMarco, 1987).

Communion

Before Christ's death, he arranged a last meal with his disciples. He took bread and wine and linked these elements with his approaching death. Jesus then instructed his disciples to repeat this meal in memory of him. The Lord's Supper, Mass, Holy Communion, or Holy Eucharist is practiced by all Christian groups but has a variety of forms and varies in significance. This can range from a simple commemoration and recognition of corporate unity to an expiatory sacrifice to take away sin. Roman Catholic couples, in particular, if in the hospital on a Sunday, should be given the option to receive this sacrament, as it is of extreme importance in the practice of their faith.

Charity

In all Christian communities, giving is seen as an intrinsic virtue. The pattern of giving was initiated in the early church and has a threefold purpose: to support the church itself, to further the work of the church, and to help poor people.

Many hospitals were built and are supported through church organizations. If a medical genetic practice is part of a hospital supported by church funding, genetic professionals need to keep in mind the religious issues of that particular group when counseling couples, as there may be practical ramifications or limitations to choice as a result. For example, in some Christian hospitals, all requests for termination of pregnancy will be denied. In others, abortions, even of known lethal conditions, need to be assessed and approved by an ethics committee.

Healing

Most Christian denominations believe strongly in the aspect of divine healing. A tradition of miracle-working has permeated the church since the time of Christ. It is important not to take away a couple's hope in the possibility of a miracle for their child, but this should be tempered with the reality of the situation. A personal example of divine intervention occurred for a Roman Catholic couple who had a fetus diagnosed with anencephaly. They did not wish to continue the pregnancy, yet did not wish to go against the moral guidelines of the Catholic Church. Coincidentally, after much prayer, pastoral consultation, and anguish, the pregnancy miscarried. The fact that the choice was taken away from this couple was significant for them.

IMPLICATIONS FOR GENETIC SERVICES

Christian beliefs and practices through history and practical applications of those beliefs to the delivery of medical genetic services have been interwoven throughout this chapter. Advocacy for special needs, diagnosis, and testing of genetic conditions are not contraindicated by Christian doctrine. Furthermore, genetic counseling that is nondirective and can uphold the belief systems of individuals is not at variance with the teaching of the Christian church. However, a number of these issues arise in medical genetic practice and can cause conflicts or moral dilemmas for Christians. They may include (1) reproductive technologies (in vitro fertilization, surrogacy, artificial insemination by donor) applied to families with a genetic disease; (2) prenatal diagnosis (amniocentesis, chorionic villus sampling, prenatal DNA testing, maternal triple screening, and ultrasound), because of the potential possibility of the termination of a fetus with a diagnosed condition; and (3) the termination of life support or refusal to treat an infant with congenital anomalies. New technologies and diagnostic techniques in and of themselves do not create the concern, but debate surrounds how information from those technologies will be used.

The basis for the conflict is that Scripture upholds the sanctity of human life. There are no direct scriptural references against reproductive technologies and abortion, but the situation is implied. The human being "created in the image of God" is called to participate in realizing the love that God wanted for humanity. Jeremiah 1:5, in a passage in which God speaks to Jeremiah, states, "Before I formed you in the womb I knew you, and before you were born I consecrated you" (New American Standard Version). Moreover, the book of Psalms 139:13 states, "For Thou didst form my inward parts; Thou didst weave me in my mother's womb" (New American Standard Version). As discussed previously, Christianity teaches love, respect, and acceptance for all humanity.

Disagreement about this issue is not simply denominational. Conservative tends to speak easily with conservative, liberal with liberal, radical with radical across denominational boundaries (Holtam, 1988). There are both absolutist and gradualist approaches within the Christian Church, and the debate is highly contentious.

The absolutist approach is the dominant view of the Eastern Orthodox and Roman Catholic churches. It is also held by the majority of conservative Protestant churches. It take the premise that life begins at conception and therefore, the status of the embryo is equated with the status of any other living human being and determines its dignity accordingly (Holtam, 1988). Therefore, with this particular emphasis on the fetus, reproductive/diagnostic technologies (e.g., abortion, amniocentesis or chorionic villus sampling) are weighed out and usually fall short if they do not lead to the healing or safeguarding of an individual (DeMarco, 1987). Even if that individual fetus is potentially handicapped/disabled, abortion is not justified because it limits "the riches of human experience."

The gradualist approach, on the other hand, believes that respect is due to the embryo at all stages, but protection of life, in the sense that a postnatal child would have it, is afforded only after some particular threshold in the pregnancy, when individuality begins to emerge. This threshold has been defined in different ways; for example, "quickening," the formation of the primitive streak, the formation of the nervous system. The emphasis of this approach is compassion for the mother balanced with responsibility to the fetus and integrally connected to the life and well-being of the woman's family (Holtam, 1988). Following from this, the use of reproductive technologies before a given threshold does not cause as much of a moral dilemma. Prenatal diagnosis, especially if done early, could be an option for a woman, and abortion would be weighed on a case-by-case basis. Abortion for a lethal condition, such as renal agenesis, or if the mother's life was in danger, could be seen as an acceptable alternative.

The termination of life-support systems in a child found postnatally to have a severe genetic condition is also an extremely difficult decision for Christian couples relating to issues of sanctity of life and acceptance of the diversity of human life. One couple made the remark, "While there is life, there is hope." However, again, each case must be weighed and a realistic perspective given to the couple. The relationship of the couple and the physician is of extreme importance. Death and dying, with accompanying loss and grief, though always a difficult situation, may be easier to accept if the couple believes that the child will be going to heaven, where there will be no more suffering.

CONCLUSION

Christians are a diverse group encompassing Catholics, Protestants, Eastern Orthodox, and a variety of other groups. The denominations share some fundamentals, but vary widely on certain issues encountered in the genetic clinical setting. Catholicism has specific guidelines for its members on a variety of issues. It forbids abortion and promotes only one means of birth control: rhythm. It also forbids all reproductive technologies. However, many American Catholics do not agree with the church's stance, especially regarding issues such as contraception. The Eastern Orthodox Church leaves many issues open to the individual's judgment, though tradition is a very strong influence. In dealing with individuals of the Protestant faith, it is wise to ask about their belief system regarding a particular issue, not to assume anything. (For one example of a Protestant group, see chapter 11, on the Amish.)

SUMMARY

—Christian doctrine does not contraindicate nondirective counseling, advocacy for special needs, or testing for genetic conditions.
—Abortion, termination of life support for severe genetic conditions, or the "do nothing" policy for lethal chromosomal conditions may be extremely difficult because of the Christian belief in the sanctity of life.

—Since Roman Catholics and many conservative Protestants believe life begins at conception, in vitro fertilization and GIFT pose dilemmas.

—For many women who become pregnant (especially before marriage) and whose child subsequently dies or is born with a birth defect, offer reassurance that this is not God's punishment. Reading of scripture or speaking with familiar clergy provides comfort to individuals in times of need.

—The church community may be a good support system when a child dies or a miscarriage occurs. Church members may help with respite care when a child has a handicap.

—Many people believe in prayer and miracles. While it is reasonable to present the medical reality, do not take away an individual's hope.

—Baptism is important to many individuals. Baptism of the infant in the womb may be necessary under certain circumstances.

—Before scheduling appointments, be aware of holy days or days of observance, especially Christmas and Easter. Seventh Day Adventists will not come to a Friday evening or Saturday clinic.

—Try not to give bad news at Christmas time. Instead, wait until the New Year, if possible.

—Marriage between cousins may be kept as a family secret, since some denominations (Catholic and Protestant) discourage, and in some cases, forbid these unions.

—Before accepting a position as a geneticist or genetic counselor in a church-affiliated institution, learn the limitations of choice for patients receiving treatment there.

—A number of nonmainstream Christian groups have very specific beliefs. For example, Jehovah's Witnesses refuse blood transfusions; therefore, intervention with children with sickle cell may require court order.

—Members of the Church of Christian Scientists believe in healing by prayer and divine law, so individuals may refuse many technological interventions, including prenatal diagnostic testing, blood tests, and autopsies.

ACKNOWLEDGMENTS

We acknowledge Margot Van Allen, M.D., and the genetic counselors in the Department of Medical Genetics, University Hospital, British Columbia, for their input, support, and encouragement.

REFERENCES

Ashley, B. M., and O'Rourke, K. D. 1989. *Health Care Ethics: A Theological Analysis,* 3d ed. St. Louis: Catholic Health Association of the United States.

Bentley, S. 1983. *Religions of Our Neighbours*. Coquitlam, Brit. Col.: Bentley West Publishing.

Bevilacqua, Cardinal Anthony. 1993. Americans with Disabilities Act: Implementation guidelines and pastoral guidelines issued by the Wisconsin Catholic Conference. *Catholic International* 4:125–27.

Brown, J. 1990. Prenatal screening in Jewish Law. *Journal of Medical Ethics* 16:75–80.

Cahill, L. S. 1989. Moral traditions, ethical language, and reproductive technologies. *Journal of Medical Philosophy* 14:497–522.

Campbell, C. S. 1990. Religion and moral meaning in bioethics. In Callahan, D., and Campbell, C. S. (eds.), *Theology, Religious Traditions, and Bioethics. Hastings Center Report* 20 (suppl.):4–10.

DeMarco, D. 1987. *In My Mother's Womb: The Catholic Church's Defense of Natural Life*. Manassas, Va.: Trinity Communications.

Fineman, R. M., Meier, G., Nye, G., and Vetrano, M. A. 1987. The religious influences on the genetic counseling process: A round table discussion. *Birth Defects* 23:154–61.

Fletcher, J. 1988. *The Ethics of Genetic Control: Ending Reproductive Roulette*. Buffalo: Prometheus Books.

Hillerbrand, H. J. 1971. The reforming spirit. In Severy, M., and Fishbein, S. L. (eds.), *Great Religions of the World*. Washington, D.C.: National Geographic Society.

Holtam, N. R. 1988. Antenatal diagnosis and the termination of pregnancy: What the churches have to say. *Journal of Inherited Metabolic Disease* 11 (suppl. 1):111–19.

Little, P. E. 1985. *Know What You Believe*. Wheaton, Ill.: Scripture Press Publications.

McCormick, R. A. 1984. *Health and Medicine in the Roman Catholic Tradition*. New York: Crossroad Publishing.

McManners, J. (ed.). 1990. *The Oxford Illustrated History of Christianity*. New York: Oxford University Press.

Sgreccia, E. 1989. Ethical issues in prenatal diagnosis and fetal therapy: A Catholic perspective. *Fetal Therapy* 4 (suppl. 1):16–27.

Smart, N. 1989. *The World's Religions: Old Traditions and Modern Transformations*. New York: Cambridge University Press.

Smith, H. 1958. *The Religions of Man*. New York: Harper & Row.

Tinley, S. T. 1987. Prenatal diagnosis in a Catholic facility. *Birth Defects* 23:262–66.

Vetrano, M. A., and Siegel, B. 1987. Clergy liaison groups. *Birth Defects* 23:206–13.

Walls, A. 1985. Christianity. In Hinnells, J. R. (ed.), *A Handbook of Living Religions,* chap. 2. New York: Viking Press.

Walton, L. 1990. Embryo research: Why the cardinal is wrong. *Journal of Medical Ethics* 16:185–86.

Whalen, J. P. 1971. The forging of Christendom. In Severy, M., and Fishbein, S. L. (eds.), *Great Religions of the World*. Washington, D.C.: National Geographic Society.

World Council of Churches. 1982. *Manipulating Life: Ethical Issues in Genetic Engineering*. Geneva: World Council of Churches.

11

Amish Culture

Clair A. Francomano, M.D.

The Old Order Amish are a socioreligious community with origins in the Anabaptist movement of the Reformation. The Anabaptists (literally, "rebaptizers") advocated adult baptism, complete separation of church and state, literal interpretation of the Bible, mutual assistance, and the principles of peace and nonresistance. Because they were neither Catholic nor Protestant, Anabaptists in sixteenth-century Europe were rejected and persecuted for their beliefs and customs. The history of martyrdom is an important aspect of the Amish cultural heritage. Many modern Amish people have demonstrated a willingness to go to jail if their beliefs conflict with secular laws.

IMMIGRATION

The followers of Jakob Ammann broke away from the original Anabaptist followers of Menno Simons (Mennonites) in the early 1690s and established a more conservative sect, which came to be known as the Amish. The Amish first settled in Pennsylvania when they arrived in the United States in the early 1700s from Germany, Switzerland, and the Alsace region of

France (McKusick, 1978). According to Hostetler (1989), there are about one hundred thirty thousand Old Order Amish in the United States. The largest settlements are in Ohio (Holmes and Wayne Counties), Indiana (Elkhart and LaGrange Counties), and Pennsylvania (Lancaster and Mifflin Counties).

The Old Order Amish are the most numerous of the Amish groups in the United States today. However, there are other closely related groups, whose views on the acceptance of modern medical technology may differ from those of the Old Order Amish. For example, the Swartzentruber Amish are extremely conservative and highly unlikely to seek modern health care for any reason. This group is among those who will not immunize their children against common childhood disorders. The New Order Amish are less conservative, and the Beachy Amish considerably more liberal in their general approach to life and to medical technology, in particular. As a rule, the more conservative Amish sects are less likely to be interested in utilizing modern medical services and technology.

Cross and McKusick (1970) studied the demographics of Amish society in Holmes County, Ohio, beginning in 1964. They found a broad-based population pyramid reflecting a relatively young population, with the majority of individuals under twenty years of age. Males outnumbered females from birth through age nine and again among those older than fifty-three, but in the intervening years the sex ratio was close to one. The median age at marriage was twenty-three years for females and twenty-four years for males, with more than one-third of the wives being older than their husbands. An estimated 7 percent of pregnancies were conceived before wedlock, but almost all couples married before the birth of the child. In 1964, the Amish community had a crude birth rate comparable to the U.S. rate in 1900, but with a 50 percent greater fertility ratio. The median number of live births to Amish women was 6.66. Birth intervals were found to be comparable to those seen in other high-fertility groups, with shorter intervals between births and a longer reproductive span among the more fertile Amish women, and a positive correlation between increasing birth order and birth intervals.

RELIGION

The Amish religion is intertwined with Amish culture: Amish life is centered around the Amish faith. The Old Order way of life is dictated by the

Ordnung, a series of rules and regulations defining how members live together (Hostetler, 1989). This document deals with all facets of life, from home furnishings to earning a livelihood. In essence, the rules and regulations embodied in the Ordnung constitute the Amish ritual of everyday life. "They provide concrete ways in which members embody the goal of loving community. Amish and Mennonite ritual takes place in the ordinary spheres of everyday life" (Cronk, 1981).

The religious communities of the Amish are interspersed throughout the landscape of the counties in which they reside. There are no central headquarters of the church. Amish communities are divided into "church districts" based on the population of a particular region. The size of these groups is dictated by the number of persons that can be accommodated in the houses and barns that host the worship services. Worship is held every other Sunday throughout the year. Every Sunday, however, is a day of contemplation and rest.

Church leaders, including ministers and bishops, are selected by lot among the men of the community. The Amish deep belief in God's will is reflected by this practice, as is the strong belief in the equality of all individuals.

The community is not only a religious community, but also a community of work, consumption, sharing of resources, and mutual aid (Hostetler, 1989). The Amish attachment to farming stems from the Creation myth in the Bible and parables that dictate stewardship of the soil: "They are to till and care for the soil with their labor and oversight" (Hostetler, 1989, p. 56). The family provides the work force for the parental farm. Offspring work on the parental farm, both to acquire the skills and knowledge to run their own farms and to provide the labor necessary to keep the farms viable.

Biblical injunctions concerning love and mutual aid are taken literally by this peace-loving people. Translation of the rule of love into everyday life prohibits unnecessary competition and rivalry.

The Amish have a strong belief in the will of God and in God's omnipresence in life's events. Illness, including genetic disease, is seen as a reflection of God's will. Intervention in the course of a disorder is often judged against the degree to which the intervention disrupts the family unit, and the likelihood that the intervention will make a significant difference in the life of a child. For example, prolonged hospitalizations are unlikely to be undertaken if the family foresees that a child will ultimately not survive in any event. Moreover, a religious proscription against the use of insurance means that high-technology modern medicine imposes a tremendous financial burden. The Amish do participate in a form of self-insurance, in which the entire community combines financial resources to support those in need of surgery or other expensive medical care. A reluctance to incur large hospital bills or to allow children perceived as mortally ill to remain in hospitals for what may be viewed as futile and expensive care may lead to a difference of opinion between health care providers and Amish families. The cultural and financial aspects of each child's illness must be carefully considered in management decisions for Amish children with genetic disorders.

An additional aspect of the strong Amish belief in God's will is an absolute proscription against the use of birth control. Likewise, artificial insemination by donor is irrelevant. Abortion is similarly prohibited, except when the life of the mother may be threatened. Prenatal diagnosis and DNA storage is therefore not an issue in this ethnic population. However, for disorders in which appropriate neonatal management depends on knowing whether or not an infant is affected, some Amish couples might consent to prenatal testing.

The entire Amish culture is deeply embedded in tradition. Every act of every day resists modernization and change. Given this, the degree to which the Amish have accepted some aspects of modern medical technology is quite surprising. Their acceptance, however, is mixed with a strong dependence on folk medicine and remedies.

Amish people live in the present rather than dwelling on the future or the past. Their way of life reflects and reveres the traditions of the past, but the rhythm of life is the gentle rhythm of the agricultural year. They plant in the spring to harvest in the fall; there is full recognition that the latter will not happen without the former. A family will conscientiously put away household items for a young woman's trousseau from the time she is a toddler, but they are not living for the future event, rather anticipating and planning for it. Reverence for family and ancestors is reflected in the meticulously kept Amish genealogies. The genealogies provide the grounding to establish where the current generations fit. The idea of one's place in the Amish culture is pervasive. An Amish man or woman walks into church services preceding and following the same two individuals for his or her entire life, because the members of a church district enter the service according to age. One Amish woman said that this provides a remarkably stabilizing sense to one's life; there is no ambiguity about one's place in the service, which never changes from the day a child is old enough to take his or her place with the adults in the religious observance.

The family is the central unit of Amish life, and very few adults who stay within the Amish fold remain unmarried. Contrary to popular belief, marriages are not arranged. The divorce rate is virtually zero; to divorce a spouse, an Amish adult would be expected to leave the community. Although unusual, nonpaternity does occur.

The Amish community is patriarchal, with the bishop (always male) being the leader of the "flock" and the father being the leader of the household. In many families, however, the influence of the mother is not to be underestimated. The father may be the spokesperson to the outside world, but decisions are often made on an equal footing between husband and wife.

The Amish eschew titles (such as Mr. or Mrs.) and prefer the use of first names. In speaking with an Amish couple about medical issues, a health care professional can more readily establish rapport by introducing him- or herself using a professional title and first name (e.g., Nurse Bill or Dr. Nancy).

Among the Old Order Amish of Lancaster County, Pennsylvania, a child's middle initial is that of the mother's unmarried name. The patriarchal nature of the society is reflected in the informal naming of individuals; Eli may have seven children who are known as Eli's John, Joseph, Aaron, and so on. His wife may be referred to as Eli's Katie. This is helpful in distinguishing among the many individuals in the community who share the same first and last names. The high frequency of inbreeding among the Amish population is reflected in a paucity of surnames (table 11.1). McKusick et al. (1964, "Distribution") discussed the use of family names to distinguish between the genetic constitutions of Amish groups in different geographic areas. For example, in Lancaster County, eight names accounted for about 80 percent of the Amish families in 1964 (McKusick, 1978).

Children play important social and economic roles in Amish society. They are considered a blessing whether or not they are healthy. Both parents care for and discipline the children. Often the older children assist in the care of younger ones, as would be expected in a culture where the average couple has seven children. Amish youngsters are taught to be stoic at a very early age; two-year-old children are expected to sit through a four-hour church service on hard benches every two weeks. Beginning at a young age, children are expected to assist with chores around the home and farm, including housework, gardening, food preservation, milking, and working in the family businesses. As a result, Amish children are exposed to the risks

Table 11.1. The Distribution (%) of Family Names in Lancaster County, Pennsylvania, and Holmes County, Ohio

Lancaster County	%	Holmes County	%
Stoltzfus (also Stoltzfoos)	23	Miller	26
King	12	Yoder	17
Fisher	12	Troyer	11
Beiler	12	Hershberger	5
Lapp	7	Raber	5
Zook	6	Schlabach	5
Esh (also Esch)	6	Weaver	4
Glick	3	Mast	4
Total 1,106 families, 1957		Total 1,611 families, 1960	

Source: Data from McKusick et al. (1964c)

of farm life, and trauma represents a significant cause of morbidity (Jones, 1990).

Amish schools are generally one-room schoolhouses shared by all grades, usually taught by an unmarried Amish woman who recently completed similar education herself. Students learn the basics of reading, writing, and arithmetic, with the older students often helping the younger ones with their assignments and reading. World geography is covered extensively. Learning is by rote, with little room for the development of independent thought or logical analysis. The educational goals are to equip the children to manage the farms, small businesses, and households of their own families as adults. When the children have completed the eighth grade, they stop attending formal classes (as affirmed by the Supreme Court decision in *Wisconsin v. Yoder et al.*) (Hostetler, 1989). At home, the girls study homemaking, and the boys study farming. They keep a diary of what they are learning and review their books with the schoolteacher once a week until their sixteenth birthday. In this way, the Amish schools satisfy the state requirements for schooling until the age of sixteen.

In the home, the Amish speak a form of German called "Pennsylvania Dutch," which Amish children learn at their parent's knee. They learn English in school, but it is rarely spoken at home. The language of the church service is a High German, entirely distinct from the German dialect spoken at home. Thus, virtually all Amish individuals are trilingual.

The Amish community has resisted the tendency toward materialism that has swept up many of the religious holidays in the secular world. Their yearly calendar centers around the agricultural seasons—times of planting and harvesting are busiest. During fall and winter, in the Lancaster County

Amish community, Tuesdays and Thursdays are wedding days, and most families will be busy with festivities. Sundays are "verboten" for medical visits, all year long.

Hostetler (1980) wrote, "The Amish believe they must be separate from the world in order to attain eternal life." As a spiritual community, they attempt to be visibly separate from the world, based on Romans 12:2, "Be not conformed to this world" (King James Version). This separation from the world is manifest in their clothing, which is plain, dark colored, and homemade. As a rule, no buttons are used, because buttons were first used as a decoration on military uniforms and so are doubly condemned for both military and worldly connotations. Women and young girls cover their heads as a sign of modesty. Men begin to grow beards (but not mustaches) at the time they marry, and many never cut them from that day forth.

The sanctity and closeness of the family is reflected in the tradition of building a *Daadi Haus* (grandfather house), or small addition, onto the family house when it is taken over by the next generation. Three or four generations of a family may thus share dwelling on the farm, each with its own private "apartment" but in close proximity to the others.

The desire to maintain a separateness from the world is manifest in the Amish avoidance of electricity, telephones, or incoming gas lines, each of which would require a physical connection to the non-Amish ("English") world. Moreover, the Amish do not own cars, trucks, or modern farm implements, although communities may differ in the extent to which farm modernization is accepted. For example, in some Amish communities the use of solid rubber tires, but not inflatable ones, on farm implements is acceptable. Some communities allow the use of a generator in the barn to power a milking apparatus, while in other communities such a generator would not be tolerated.

Animals play a large role in the community structure, as they did in eighteenth- and nineteenth-century agricultural America. Horses provide farm assistance and power horse-and-buggy transportation. Cows provide milk for drinking and for dairy products, and are butchered for beef. Chickens are grown for eggs and meat.

Almost all Amish homes have a garden to provide fruits and vegetables for the family. Vegetables are cooked fresh in the summer and fall, then canned or otherwise preserved for the winter. However, the paucity of arable land in many Amish communities is compelling some young couples to move to remote settlements in Canada and the Midwest, thus breaking up the integrity of the family unit, which has been sacrosanct over the centuries of Amish life in America.

COMMUNICATION

Because English is a second language for Amish people, their oral English communication may come across as stilted or awkward. It is important for health care professionals to understand that this in no way reflects a lack of intelligence or literacy. Informality in forms of address will ease the development of rapport. Discussions are best held face to face, as the Amish value face-to-face communication (Waltman, 1996). Maintaining eye contact and seeking to establish common ground on an emotionally difficult discussion will help keep the lines of communication open. Most Amish people will engage in a minimal amount of small talk before discussing the issue at hand, but only enough to be sociable. It is well to allow a reasonable amount of physical space between the Amish patient and the health care professional during an interview, avoiding physical contact, especially between individuals of different genders, except as needed for physical examination.

Idioms can present problems on occasion. One Amish woman told the author that Amish people, in general, have an aversion to referring to their offspring as "kids." She averred that goats have kids, while humans have children.

In addressing an Amish couple, health care professionals should speak slowly and in a soft tone of voice, but in a conversational way, without appearing condescending. Both members of the couple should be addressed directly, but one should expect responses from the father. Diagrams and written illustrations will assist in communication. Since the Amish do not watch television or go to movie theaters, brochures and written communications are more in keeping with their culture than videotapes for transmitting educational information.

Stoicism is an important part of the Amish culture. Neither children nor adults readily admit to physical or emotional pain. Because of their rock-solid belief in the will of God and the continuity of life in the hereafter, death is viewed as a relief of suffering and a "passing over" to a better place. Waltman (1996) cited the reaction of an Amish acquaintance, whose wife died suddenly of a myocardial infarction: "I guess it was just her time."

Kaiser (1986) wrote of a couple whose infant son was born with a hereditary form of microcephaly, and whose death she attended when the child was about seven months old: the family thanked her for not doing anything to prolong his life and his pain.

BELIEFS ABOUT HEALTH

The *Budget,* a weekly newspaper published by and for the Amish, contains many reports about health and illness. Home remedies or patent medicines are often the first line of defense against unexplained symptoms. Almost any issue of the *Budget* will contain ads for mail-order remedies to cure common disorders, including arthritis, lack of energy, bowel dysfunction, skin complaints, and other ailments. A column called "Information Please" allows readers to exchange home remedies. Waltman (1996) cited one column recommending, for the treatment of boils, drinking black walnut leaf tea, eating raisins, or adding burdock root to drinking water.

Amish people are also prone to consulting nontraditional medical therapists. The Amish folk practitioner of the "braucha," or pow-wow, is less prevalent today than thirty years ago, but such persons still are found in Amish communities. These individuals, whose training is an oral tradition from generation to generation, use quotations from the Bible, charms such as a raw egg or a chicken, or physical manipulation to treat physical complaints. Other nontraditional practitioners who may be consulted include reflexologists, who believe that many human ills may be solved by appropriate manipulation of the feet. An Amish kitchen in the home of a family using such a practitioner will often have a detailed chart of the foot, illustrating the parts of the body regulated by the manipulation of each region. Massage therapists and chiropractors are other frequently consulted nontraditional practitioners.

An understanding of the Amish approach to health care requires exploration of their cultural definitions of health and illness. Hostetler (1980, p. 313) observed that "the Amish emphasize hard work, and for them, a healthy person is one who has a good appetite, looks physically well, and can do rigorous physical labor." Illness is defined not by subjective symptoms but by the degree of one's ability to perform expected tasks at home or at work. For this reason, medical care may not be sought until an illness has become incapacitating.

The Amish system of education precludes training an Amish youth to be a traditional health care professional. The higher education necessary for such training would require leaving the Amish community. Moreover, although the educational system provided by the Amish amply prepares their youth for the skills required to run a farm, a small business, or a household, the level of sophistication with regard to biological and medical principles is low. Therefore, the successful health practitioner in the Amish community will take the time to explain, in very basic language, the perceived medical problem and the proposed approach or solution. Tolerance of alternative health care choices, including folk medicine practitioners and home remedies, is advocated, as far as they are perceived to be benign in effect.

The Amish faith does not prohibit the use of modern medicine. Blood transfusions, anesthesia and surgery, biopsies, blood tests, as well as modern technological equipment in a hospital, are all condoned and used by members of Amish communities. Among the more conservative Amish groups, there are those who would not utilize modern medical practices, but they represent a small minority of the Amish people.

However, cultural and financial aspects of Amish life may interfere with the utilization of modern health care services. These barriers include the absence of health insurance, the logistical problems imposed by distance from a large medical center, and the proscription against automobiles. A trip that seems trivial if traveling by automobile may take most of the day in a horse and buggy. This problem has been mitigated somewhat in recent years by the use of "drivers." These are usually local men, often of the less conservative Mennonite faith, who make a living or supplement their income by driving cars or vans to transport Amish people over distances that would be prohibitive by horse and buggy. Although the actual trip is more easily accomplished in this way, a prolonged hospitalization of any member of the family imposes extreme hardship on the functioning family unit, which depends on the presence of mother, father, and children to operate smoothly.

Amish people do not participate in commercial insurance or government assistance programs. This reflects their desire not to be dependent on persons outside their own faith. Instead, they have established a form of self-insurance for property and health care which assists in covering the costs of modern medical care. Participating families make regular financial contributions. Because of recent astronomical increases in the costs of health care, such funds may be readily depleted by a single prolonged hospitalization. For this reason, any decision to enter into a form of treatment likely to result in a large medical bill is made with the knowledge that the resources used to support such therapy may not be there when another person needs them. Hence, medical decisions may be made keeping in mind the greater good of the community, as opposed to that of the individual.

If self-insurance funds are depleted, additional contributions are sought on a voluntary basis from both Amish and non-Amish sources. The Rainbow of Hope Foundation, a cooperative effort between Amish and non-Amish people in the Holmes County, Ohio, region, was established to aid any family in the area with costs incurred in the care of an infant or child with a catastrophic illness (Waltman, 1996).

In general, the Amish life style is conducive to good health. Amish men, more than Amish women, are exposed to rigorous exercise in their work around the farms. Amish families eat well, and religious prohibitions against the use of tobacco, alcohol, and drugs (for other than medicinal purposes) are usually followed (Fuchs et al., 1990).

In the Amish view, death is part of the cycle of life, as much a part of the rhythm of things as the winter following the fall. Terminally ill family members are cared for at home by loving family members with strong community emotional support and assistance around the home and farm. Sudden death, accidental death, and death resulting from genetic or other chronic disorders are all seen as reflecting God's will.

Maternal and child health practices are inextricably intertwined with the fabric of the Amish religion and culture. Prenatal care is often sought early in the first pregnancy. However, subsequent pregnancies may not come to medical attention until as late as the third trimester, especially if the mother is feeling well. Here again, the pregnancy is viewed as representative of God's will, and as an integral part of the natural cycle of life. The idea that medical care is necessary for the management of a pregnancy is foreign to this view of reproduction.

An Amish midwife, nurse midwife, medical doctor, or doctor of osteopathy may attend the delivery. Many Amish couples prefer the delivery to take place at home; this provides the least possible disruption of family life. A survey of Wayne County, Ohio, Amish found that "first deliveries and those with predictable medical complications were the childbirths most likely to occur in a hospital" (Heikes, 1985). Recently, physicians attending many Amish couples opened birthing centers in Holmes and Geauga Counties, in Ohio. The birthing center at Mount Eaton, which opened in 1985, provides a homelike atmosphere where labor, delivery, and postpartum care are all accomplished in the patient's room. Only low-risk, "normal" deliveries are scheduled at this site. In keeping with Amish cultural expectations, the rooms do not have televisions or telephones. Lamps simulating the gas lamps used in Amish homes have been installed in the birthing rooms to provide a more "homey" atmosphere. (Real gas lamps could not be used because of fire codes.) Overnight accommodations are available for the father, as well as the buggy horses. As a rule, mother and baby are discharged home after twenty-four hours.

Some hospitals in regions where there are large Amish populations have also instituted the birthing center concept, attempting to accommodate the Amish desire for the mother and child to be together from the moment of birth and to return to the family fold as quickly as possible, as well as to minimize the expense related to labor, delivery, and postnatal care.

Unless there is a medical reason to avoid breastfeeding, virtually all Amish babies are breastfed. Circumcision is not a universal practice, and the decision regarding circumcision is made by the parents and communicated to the health care providers, usually by the father.

The prohibition against participation in governmental aid programs is not rigid, and may be overlooked if a child with special needs is born and may benefit from supplemental income programs for handicapped children or programs that provide financial assistance for the medical care of such youngsters. The parental decision to participate in such programs may need to be made in consultation with the elders of the church community or perhaps the bishop.

The acceptance of immunization practices varies. The majority of "mainstream" Amish people vaccinate their children (Heikes, 1985). However, the more conservative sects are less likely to participate in immunization programs. Waltman (1996) speculated that the objections to immunizations are either that they are too modern or that they are too similar to insurance. She cited Guyther (1979), who proposed that some Amish parents object to the use of immunizations on the grounds that, in allowing one's child to be vaccinated, "one may be lacking in the faith that God will protect, and consequently is hedging his bet that the child will not contract a serious communicable disease."

An Amish couple may choose not to prolong the life of an infant affected by a genetic disorder if they perceive that the intervention will only prolong the child's suffering and not alter the inevitable outcome. This approach may put an Amish couple at odds with the staff of a modern intensive care nursery, who are trained to "do everything." Attempts by hospital staff to gain custody of a child to pursue a more aggressive course of therapy than is desired by the family may be successful for the case at hand, but will almost certainly alienate both the family of the child and much of the rest of the community, who will avoid subsequent births at the hospital that undertakes such litigation.

Miller and Schwartz (1992) studied the attitudes toward genetic testing of Amish families with cystic fibrosis, comparing them to Mennonite, Hutterite, and "English" families with the same disorder. After having a child with cystic fibrosis and learning the recurrence of the risk, 72 percent of the Amish couples were uncertain as to whether they would change their planned family size. Eighty-six percent did not approve of or were uncertain about the use of prenatal diagnosis, while the couples were evenly split between wanting to know and not wanting to know the results of carrier testing for their children. The investigators speculated that some Amish families might use the results of carrier testing to influence the selection of mates for their carrier children. The majority of couples were uncertain as to whether carriers should be allowed to marry carriers. One hundred percent of Amish couples were either opposed to or uncertain about elective abortion of prenatally diagnosed fetuses affected by cystic fibrosis.

IMPLICATIONS FOR GENETIC SERVICES

Geneticists have interacted with the Amish population over the years, both to provide genetic services and to advance medical knowledge concerning the genetic disorders that are more common among the Amish than the non-Amish population. The Amish are an outstanding population for genetic studies for several reasons:

1. The high degree of inbreeding has resulted in the presence of a large number of recessive disorders, many of which were unrecognized outside of the Amish population.
2. The community is a closed community. Members may leave, but outsiders join the community extremely rarely.
3. Amish genealogies are extensive and meticulously maintained. One of the most extensive Lancaster County genealogies, the *Fisher Book* (Beiler, 1988), is now available on computer through the laboratory of Wilma Bias, Ph.D., at Johns Hopkins University. This resource enables the tracking of common ancestors and "loops" of inbreeding in a much more efficient manner than was possible in the precomputer era.

McKusick, Hostetler, and Egeland (1964) cited the following additional aspects of Amish society as advantageous for genetic studies:

1. The population is relatively well nourished, and infectious diseases are not likely to confound the interpretation of findings.

2. In general, standards of medical care are high.

3. The uniformity of socioeconomic status reduces this source of variability in the population.

4. The average level of consanguinity is high, leading to a high frequency of rare recessive disorders.

5. Family size is large—an average of 6.66 children per couple.

6. The population is immobile because of its agrarian life style. (As already mentioned, this has changed somewhat in the last decade, but it is still true that large kindreds are available for study in a limited geographic area.)

7. The Amish are clannish and are likely to be aware of illness in extended branches of their families.

There are drawbacks, too. Obtaining written consent presents a problem in the Amish community. The Amish believe that their word is as good as their bond. Requiring written consent suggests, in this culture, that the health care professional does not trust the word of the Amish patient or subject. At Johns Hopkins University, where numerous research projects related to the genetic disorders found among Amish people have originated over the years, this has been a particularly difficult issue with the Joint Committee on Clinical Investigation, the committee for the protection of human subjects. Wilma Bias, Professor of Medicine, is an immunogeneticist who has coordinated most of the investigative work from Johns Hopkins among the Lancaster County Amish over the last twenty years. She invited an Amish bishop from Lancaster County to a meeting of the Joint Committee on Clinical Investigation to present the case against requiring written consent from Amish subjects in genetic studies; the committee then granted permission for the studies to be done without written consent. Field workers document that they have read to the participants a standardized form listing the reasons for a proposed study and the potential risks and benefits. A list of subjects is then kept in the immunogenetics logbook for each day of field work, with the field worker signing a form stating that oral informed consent was obtained from each subject.

In general, the Amish will not allow autopsies on deceased family members. There are probably several reasons behind this reluctance. An Amish family will usually express the concern that the deceased has "suffered enough" and need not be subjected to the perceived indignity and mutilation of autopsy. The tradition is of rapid burial, usually within three days after death, and often the family will be concerned that autopsy will delay the availability of the body for burial. Furthermore, a lack of medical sophistication limits the degree to which the bereaved family may understand the potential value of an autopsy to furthering medical knowledge. However, as is generally the case, the existence of a longstanding, strong, and mutually trusting relationship between the physician and the family may overcome these barriers. Several Amish families have arranged for deceased members to be transported from Lancaster County to Johns Hopkins in Baltimore because of longstanding relationships with Victor McKusick, M.D., and other geneticists who persuaded them of the value of the autopsy.

Another taboo of importance to professionals interested in genetic disorders is the prohibition against taking photographs. This is in keeping with the biblical injunction against making graven images. Some families will allow photographs to be taken of their children if they are assured that the pictures will be used for medical purposes only. However, many of the more conservative Amish families are uncomfortable with photographs under any circumstances. The health care professional is wise not to push too hard on this issue. If the family feels pressured, rapport is lost and any further opportunity, either to provide genetic services or to pursue further investigation, is imperiled.

Adoption of an orphan within the family or community is acceptable, but even for an infertile couple, adoption outside the community is never done. To do so would not be accepting of "God's will."

Amish couples will often report that they are not related if the common ancestor was more than three generations in the past. A search through genealogical records or a carefully documented pedigree going back three or four generations may be necessary to establish consanguinity and the coefficient thereof.

Several resources are available to geneticists seeking genealogical information about Amish families. The *Fisher Book* (Beiler, 1988) is a genealogical registry compiling the vital events of all individuals descended from several of the pioneer families who settled in Lancaster County in the 1700s. Each nuclear family has a unique identifying number, referred to as the *Fisher Book* number. The entry for each nuclear family contains: (1) the names of husband and wife; (2) their dates of birth, marriage, and death; (3) the *Fisher Book* numbers of their parents; and (4) the names of all children. For children who never marry, or who die in childhood, dates of birth and death are given in the entry of their parents. Only the *Fisher Book* numbers of married children, who have their own unique numbers, are given in the parental entries. The most recent edition, the third, was revised and updated by a committee of Fisher descendants, and contains information up to 1988.

The *Lancaster County Directory* provides supplementary information to the *Fisher Book.* This directory represents a private population census, with a description of all Amish families living in Lancaster County and neighboring Amish communities. Unlike the *Fisher Book,* the directory lists only households with living members. The *Lancaster County Directory* contains maps that indicate each of the church districts and locate homes of each Amish member of the district noted on the maps. These maps have proven invaluable for finding families in the Lancaster County countryside. Similar directories are available for the Amish communities in Holmes and Geauga counties, Ohio, and LaGrange County, Indiana.

The *Diary* is a national Amish journal, published monthly since 1969. Reporters in each of the Amish communities across the nation communicate data from their own region on monthly listings of births, deaths, and marriages; names of parents of all who marry; location of residence for all births and deaths; information on stillbirths; and details on the circumstances surrounding a death.

Khoury (1985) studied patterns of inbreeding in Lancaster County, and the effects of inbreeding on prereproductive mortality (defined as death before age twenty years). Despite the Amish prohibition on first cousins or first cousins once-removed marrying, Khoury found that the levels of inbreeding have risen significantly over time, with the average inbreeding coefficient at the time of his study slightly less than the equivalent of a second-cousin marriage. Ninety-eight percent of all marriages had some demonstrable degree of consanguinity. These findings were somewhat surprising. Several of our Amish contacts in Lancaster County reported that since McKusick began his genetic studies in the early 1960s, there has been an increasing awareness of the possible detrimental effects of "marrying close," and that as a result young people have been sent to distant Amish communities in attempts to find mates who are not as closely related.

In his longitudinal study, Khoury (1985) found that the offspring inbreeding coefficient was an independent predictor of prereproductive mortality: the higher the coefficient, the higher the relative risk of mortality. In addition, high coefficients were associated with higher risks of multiple deaths in the same sibship. His data showed that inbreeding accounts for about 40 percent of all prereproductive deaths in the present Amish population.

Table 11.2. Mendelian Disorders in Amish People

Disorder	Population	Reference
Ellis-van Creveld syndrome	Lancaster Co.	McKusick at al., 1964b; Murdoch et al., 1964
Recessive deafness	Lancaster Co.	Mengle et al., 1969
Ataxia-telangiectasia	Holmes Co.	Ginter and Tallapragada, 1975; Rary et al., 1975
Weill-Marchesani syndrome	Lancaster Co.	Scott, 1969
Mast syndrome	Holmes Co.	Cross and McKusick, 1967a
Troyer syndrome	Holmes Co.	Cross and McKusick, 1967b
Pyruvate kinase deficiency	Mifflin Co., Pa.	Bowman et al., 1964; Oski et al., 1969
Phenylketonuria	Elkhart Co., Ind.	Martin et al., 1963
Limb-girdle muscular dystrophy	Indiana	Jackson and Stehler, 1968
Asymmetric septal hypertrophy	Indiana	Bingle et al., 1975
Cartilage hair hypoplasia	Lancaster and Holmes Co.	McKusick et al., 1965; Lux et al., 1970
Hydrometrocolpos	Lancaster Co.	McKusick et al., 1964a
Intrahepatic cholestasis	Lancaster Co.	Clayton et al., 1969; Linarelli et al., 1969
Amish albinism	Daviess Co., Ind.	Nance et al., 1970
Adducted thumbs syndrome	Daviess Co., Ind.	Christian et al., 1971
Stoltzfus blood group	Lancaster Co.	Bias et al., 1969
Hairy elbows syndrome	Lancaster Co.	Beighton, 1970
Oculocerebral syndrome with hypopigmentation	Holmes Co.	Cross et al., 1967
Bipolar affective disorder	Lancaster Co.	Egeland et al., 1987; Pauls et al., 1991; Law et al., 1992
Glutaric adicuria type I	Lancaster Co.	Morton et al., 1991
Hemophilia B	Western Pa.	Ketterling et al., 1991
Cystic fibrosis	New York State	Watkins et al., 1986; Miller et al., 1992
Familial hypothyroidism	Holmes Co.	Cross et al., 1968

Source: Abstracted, in part, from McKusick (1978)

Table 11.2 lists Mendelian disorders reported among Amish people, the community in which they were described, and relevant references. Recent studies have also focused on more common, presumably oligogenic disorders, including manic-depressive illness (Egeland et al., 1987; Pauls et al., 1991; Law et al., 1992), breast cancer (Gordon, 1991), and obesity (Stunkard, 1991).

CONCLUSION

Religion is the guide for the Amish people. It dominates their whole life, and in the past they have suffered persecution for their values and beliefs. The core unit of Amish life is the family, and children have a key role in society. Children are cherished for themselves whether or not they have a disability. The Amish community works to help its members for the good of society. The culture is traditional and most modern technology is resisted. The Amish way of life reflects respect for the past, and the rhythm of life is like the seasons: There is a time to be born and a time to die.

SUMMARY

—Provider introductions should be informal—"Dr. Nancy," "Nurse Bill"—rather than using formal titles.

—Maintain eye contact, speak in a soft voice, and maintain distance from the Amish patient.

—Begin with "small talk," but keep it brief.

—Although the father is the head of the household, decisions are made on an equal footing between husband and wife—address concerns and direct information directly to both parents.

—Birth control, abortion, DNA storage, and artificial insemination by donor are irrelevant because of the strong belief in "God's will."

—Carrier screening may be unacceptable, but the communities are now aware of the high degree of consanguinity and are looking at other Anabaptist communities for marital partner possibilities.

—Photographing a patient is usually not acceptable, but may be permitted if it is explained to be necessary in obtaining a second opinion or for establishing a medical diagnosis.

—Do not schedule clinics on Sundays, or Tuesdays and Thursdays (wedding days) in the fall.

—Consent for autopsy is usually declined.

—Plan ahead. Send written confirmation of an appointment well in advance. Telephone, electronic mail, and fax machines are not used in Amish communities. Follow-up letters are a good means of communication.

—The Amish have no commercial or government-sponsored health insurance, which may influence the decision to undergo extensive diagnostic testing.

—Written consent is not well understood. One's word is accepted within Amish communities. Two witnesses may need to give written testimony of oral consent.

—Printed visual aids may be helpful in counseling sessions.

—Immunizations are often performed, but may be declined in more conservative communities. However, such families may consent to immunizing children with special needs (e.g., immune disorders or life-threatening conditions).

—Most Amish people are trilingual, though English is not the primary language and therefore may not be fluent. Do not interpret this as a lack of literacy.

—Try to avoid the use of slang. Children, for example, should always be called by name and never referred to as "kids" (kids are understood to be baby goats).

—Tolerance for "nontraditional" and folk medicine will assist in achieving acceptance of the modern health practitioner by the Amish family.

REFERENCES

Beighton, P. 1970. Familial hypertrichosis cubiti: The hairy elbows syndrome. *Journal of Medical Genetics* 7:158–60.

Beiler, K. (ed.). 1988. *Fisher Family History*. Lancaster, Pa.: EB's Quality Printing.

Bias, W. B., Light-Orr, J. K., Krevans, J. R., Humphrey, R. L., Hamill, P. V. V., Cohen, B. H., and McKusick, V. A. 1969. The Stoltzfus blood group: A new polymorphism in man. *American Journal of Human Genetics* 21:552–58.

Bingle, G. J., Dillon, J., and Hurwitz, R. 1975. Asymmetric septal hypertrophy in a large Amish kindred. *Clinical Genetics* 7:255–61.

Bowman, H. S., McKusick, V. A., and Dronamraju, K. R. 1965. Pyruvate kinase deficient hemolytic anemia in an Amish isolate. *American Journal of Human Genetics* 17:1–8.

Christian, J. C., Andrews, P. A., Conneally, P. M., and Muller, J. 1971. The adducted thumbs syndrome: An autosomal recessive disease with arthrogryposis, dysmyelination, craniostenosis, and cleft palate. *Clinical Genetics* 2:95–103.

Clayton, R. J., Iber, F. L., Ruebner, B. H., and McKusick, V. A. 1969. Byler disease: Fatal familial intrahepatic cholestasis in an Amish kindred. *American Journal of Diseases of Children* 117:112–24.

Cronk, S. L. 1981. Gelassenheit: The rites of the redemptive process in Old Order Amish and Old Order Mennonite communities. *Mennonite Quarterly Review* 55:5–44.

Cross, H. E., and McKusick, V. A. 1967a. The Mast syndrome: A recessively inherited form of presenile dementia with motor disturbances. *Archives of Neurology* 16:1–13.

———. 1967b. The Troyer syndrome: A recessive form of spastic paraplegia with distal muscle wasting. *Archives of Neurology* 16:473–85.

———. 1970. Amish demography. *Social Biology* 17:83–101.

Cross, H. E., McKusick, V. A., and Breen, W. 1967. A new oculocerebral syndrome with hypopigmentation. *Journal of Pediatrics* 70:398–406.

Cross, H. E., Hollander, C. S., Rimoin, D. L., and McKusick, V. A. 1968. Familial agoitrous cretinism accompanied by muscular hypertrophy. *Pediatrics* 41:413–20.

Egeland, J. A., Gerhard, D. S., Pauls, D. L., Sussex, J. N., Kidd, K. K., Allen, C. R., Hostetter, A. M., and Housman, D. E. 1987. Bipolar affective disorders linked to DNA markers on chromosome 11. *Nature* 325:783–87.

Fuchs, J. A., Levinson, R. M., Stoddard, R. R., Mullet, M. E., and Jones, D. H. 1990. Health risk factors among the Amish: Results of a survey. *Health Education Quarterly* 17:197–211.

Ginter, D. N., and Tallapragada, R. 1975. Ataxia-telangiectasia. In Bergsma, D. (ed.), *Malformation Syndromes,* pp. 408–9. Birth Defects Original Article Series, no. 11. Washington, D.C.: March of Dimes.

Gordon, G. 1991. Personal communication.

Guyther, J. R. 1979. Medical attitudes of the Amish. *Maryland State Medical Journal* 28:40–41.

Heikes, J. K. 1985. Differences among the Old Order Amish of Wayne County, Ohio, and their use of health care services. Master's thesis, Ohio State University.

Hostetler, J. 1980. *Amish Society.* 3d ed. Baltimore: Johns Hopkins University Press.

———. 1989. *Amish Roots.* Baltimore: Johns Hopkins University Press.

Jackson, C. E., and Strehler, D. A. 1968. Limb-girdle muscular dystrophy: Clinical manifestations and detection of preclinical disease. *Pediatrics* 41:495–502.

Jones, M. W. 1990. A study of trauma in an Amish community. *Journal of Trauma* 30:899–902.

Kaiser, G. H. 1986. *Dr. Frau, a Woman Doctor among the Amish.* Intercourse, Pa.: Good Books.

Ketterling, R. P., Bottema, C. D. K., Koeberl, D. D., Ii, S., and Sommer, S. S. 1991. $T^{296} \rightarrow M$, A common mutation causing mild Hemophilia B in the Amish and others: Founder effect, variability in factor IX activity assays, and rapid carrier detection. *Human Genetics* 87:333–37.

Khoury, M. 1985. Inbreeding and prereproductive mortality in the Old Order Amish. Ph.D. diss., Johns Hopkins University.

Law, A., Richard, C. W., III, Cottingham, R. W., Jr., Lathrop, G. M., Cox, D. R., and Myers, R. M. 1992. Genetic linkage analysis of bipolar affective disorder in an Old Order Amish pedigree. *Human Genetics* 88:562–68.

Linarelli, L. G., Williams, C. N., and Phillips, M. J. 1972. Byler's disease: Fatal intrahepatic cholestasis. *Journal of Pediatrics* 81:484–92.

Lux, S. E., Johnston, R. B., Jr., August, C. S., Say, B., Penchaszadeh, V. B., Rosen, F. S., and McKusick, V. A. 1970. Chronic neutropenia and abnormal cellular immunity in cartilage-hair hypoplasia. *New England Journal of Medicine* 282:234–36.

McKusick, V. A. 1978. *Medical Genetic Studies of the Amish.* Baltimore: Johns Hopkins University Press.

McKusick, V. A., and Cross, H. E. 1966. Ataxia-telangiectasia and Swiss-type agammaglobulinemia: Two genetic disorders of the immune mechanism in related Amish sibships. *Journal of the American Medical Association* 195:739–45.

McKusick, V. A., Hostetler, J. A., and Egeland, J. A. 1964. Genetic studies of the Amish: Background and potentialities. *Bulletin of the Johns Hopkins Hospital* 115:203–22.

McKusick, V. A., Bauer, R. L., Koop, C. E., and Scott, R. B. 1964. Hydrometrocolpos as a simply inherited malformation. *Journal of the American Medical Association* 189:813–16.

McKusick, V. A., Egeland, J. A., Eldridge, R., and Krusen, D. E. 1964. Dwarfism in the Amish: I. The Ellis–van Creveld syndrome. *Bulletin of the Johns Hopkins Hospital* 115:306–36.

McKusick, V. A., Hostetler, J. A., Egeland, J. A., and Eldridge, R. 1964. The distribution of certain genes in the Old Order Amish. *Cold Spring Harbor Symposium on Quantitative Biology* 29:99–114.

McKusick, V. A., Eldridge, R., Hostetler, J. A., Ruangwit, U., and Egeland, J. A. 1965. Dwarfism in the Amish: II. Cartilage-hair hypoplasia. *Bulletin of the Johns Hopkins Hospital* 116:285–326.

Martin, P. H., Davis, L., and Askew, D. 1963. High incidence of phenylketonuria in an isolated Indiana community. *Journal of Indiana State Medical Association* 56:997–99.

Mengel, M. C., Konigsmark, B. W., and McKusick, V. A. 1969. Two types of congenital recessive deafness. *Eye Ear Nose Throat Monthly* 48:301–5.

Miller, S. R., and Schwartz, R. H. 1992. Attitudes toward genetic testing of Amish, Mennonite, and Hutterite families with cystic fibrosis. *American Journal of Public Health* 82:236–42.

Morton, D. H., Bennett, M. J., Seargeant, L. E., Nichter, C. A., and Kelley, R. I. 1991. Glutaric aciduria type I: A common cause of episodic encephalopathy and spastic paralysis in the Amish of Lancaster County, Pennsylvania. *American Journal of Medical Genetics* 41:89–95.

Murdoch, J. L., and Walker, B. A. 1969. Ellis–van Creveld syndrome. *The Clinical Delineation of Birth Defects: IV. Skeletal Dysplasias,* pp. 279–88. New York: National Foundation March of Dimes.

Nance, W. E., Jackson, C. E., and Witcop, C. J., Jr. 1970. Amish albinism: A distinctive autosomal recessive phenotype. *American Journal of Human Genetics* 22:579–86.

Oski, F. A., and Bowman, H. 1969. A low Km phosphoenolpyruvate mutant in the Amish with red cell pyruvate kinase deficiency. *British Journal of Haematology* 17:289–97.

Pauls, D. L., Gerhard, D. S., Lacy, L. G., Hostetter, A. M., Allen, C. R., Bland, S. D., LaBuda, M. C., and Egeland, J. A. 1991. Linkage of bipolar affective disorders to markers on chromosome 11p is excluded in a second lateral extension of Amish Pedigree 110. *Genomics* 11:730–36.

Rary, J. M., Bender, M. A., and Kelly, T. E. 1975. A 14 / 14 marker chromosome lymphocyte clone in ataxia telangiectasia. *Journal of Heredity* 66:33–35.

Scott, C. I. 1969. Weill-Marchesani syndrome. In *The Clinical Delineation of Birth Defects: II. Malformation Syndromes,* pp. 238–40. New York: National Foundation March of Dimes.

Stunkard, J. 1991. Personal communication.

Van-der-Burgt, I., Haraldsson, A., Oosterwijk, J. C., van Essen, A. J., Weemaes, C., and Hamel, B. 1991. Cartilage hair hypoplasia, metaphyseal chondrodysplasia type McKusick: Description of seven patients and review of the literature. *American Journal of Medical Genetics* 41:371–80.

Waltman, G. H. 1996. Amish health care beliefs and practices. In Julia, M. (ed.), *Multicultural Awareness in the Health Care Profession.* Boston: Allyn & Bacon.

Watkins, P. C., Schwartz, R., Hoffman, N., Stanislovitis, P., Doherty, R., and Klinger, K. 1986. A linkage study of cystic fibrosis in extended multigenerational pedigrees. *American Journal of Human Genetics* 39:735–43.

Zook, L., and Waltman, G. H. N.d. Membership and mutual aid: The Amish community as case example. Unpublished paper.

12

Jewish Culture in North America

Mark A. Greenstein, M.D., and
Bruce A. Bernstein, Ph.D.

Ethnoculturally sensitive genetic counseling for Jewish individuals implies attention to two sets of issues associated with "Jewishness" or "Jews." These terms can refer to an individual's cultural and religious orientations—the beliefs, attitudes, and customary practices that affect daily routines and the way in which life decisions are made. In addition, the terms *Jewish* and *Jews* are used to describe an ethnic group—a people with a common biological background sharing cultural traditions. Genetic counseling assumes importance in this context, since a variety of specific conditions, or particular haplotypes for these, occur more frequently among people of Jewish descent generally or among people from Jewish ancestry of a particular geographic area (tables 12.1 and 12.2).

It can be challenging for a genetics professional to identify the salient cultural or genealogical issues for an individual. From a cultural perspective, a wide variety of people identify themselves as being Jewish or of Jewish descent. While many scholarly discussions review the issue of who is Jewish and well-defined religious definitions exist, the matter remains ambiguous in practice.[1] It might seem easiest to include as Jews simply those who identify themselves as Jewish; however, this may exclude those who do not practice an organized religion or participate in Jewish cultural tradi-

Table 12.1. More Commonly Recognized Genetic Diseases with Increased Incidence in Jewish Populations

Disease	McKusick #	Probable or Known Pattern of Inheritance	Jewish Populations/ Comments
Bloom syndrome	210900	AR	32% of cases, Ashkenazi; Bloom syndrome registry
Familial cysautonomia	223900	AR	Ashkenazi (Polish)
Gaucher disease, Type I (and variants)	230800.0007ff	AR	Ashkenazi
Mucolipidosis IV	252650	AR	Ashkenazi, S. Poland
Niemann-Pick disease	257200	AR	Ashkenazi
Tay Sachs disease	272800	AR	Ashkenazi
Torsion dystonia	224500	AR	Ashkenazi (higher) and Sephardi

Sources: Mourant, Kopec, and Domaniewska-Sobczak (1978); Goodman (1979); McKusick (1994)
Note: AR, autosomal recessive

tions, but still require genetic counseling based on their ethnic heritage. The latter might include individuals whose ancestors converted to other religions but who retain the carrier frequency or risk characteristic of specific Jewish groups.

Genetic counselors must take care to avoid confounding the concept of Jews as an ethnic group with the inaccurate notion of Jews as a separate "race." The world's Jewish population is clearly composed of people of different races. The concept of Jews as a "race" may also carry disturbing echoes of the Holocaust, when "Jewishness" was cast as a racial issue.

It is difficult even within Judaism to reach consensus on the meaning or importance of practices within the various levels of orthodoxy. Accordingly, this chapter should be viewed as only an introduction to and one perspective of a complex subject. Readers are encouraged to consult more detailed discussions, both specific to genetics (especially Goodman, 1979; Mourant, Kopec, and Domaniewska-Sobczak, 1978; Bonne-Tamir and Adam, 1992) and concerning Jewish practice and culture in general (e.g., Kolatch, 1981, 1985).

Table 12.2. Additional Genetic Diseases of Note in Jewish Populations

Disease	McKusick #	Probable or Known Pattern of Inheritance	Jewish Populations / Comments
Abetalipoproteinemia	200100	AR	Jews, unspecified
Adrenal hyperplasia	202010	AR	Esp. N. African
Adrenal hyperplasia III, nonclassic and cryptic	201910	AR	Ashkenazi. Generally mild
Afibringenemia, congenital	202400	AR	In consanguineous pairings within Jewish communities in Israel
Ataxia-telangiectasia	208900	AR	Sephardi
Canavan disease	271900	AR	Ashkenazi
Cataract-mental retardation-hypogonadism	212720	AR	2 of 3 cases of Jewish descent, 1 Ashkenazi, 1 Sephardi
Cerebral cholesterinosis	213700	AR	Moroccan (Sephardi)
Chronic familial neutropenia	162700	AD	Yemenite and Ethiopian
Cohen syndrome	216550	AR	Ashkenazi
Complement C_7 deficiency	217070	AR	Sephardi (Moroccan, Yemenite, Tunisian)
Creutzfeldt-Jakob disease	123400	AD	Libyan, with possible increase in Egyptian and Tunisian
Cystic disease of lungs	219600	AR	Oriental, esp. Yemenite
Cystic fibrosis	219700	AR	No increase above most Caucasian, but increased variability of haplotypes
Cystinosis, early onset or infantile	219800	AR	N. African
Cystinuria (types I and II)	220100	AR	Libyan
Dalmation hypouricemia	220150	AR	Sephardi and Iraqi
Ectopic thyroid with hypothyroidism	225250	AR	Nonconsanguineous Ashkenzai
Familial deafness	nonspecific	AR	N. African, esp. Moroccan
Familial Mediterranean fever	249100	AR	Sephardi
Familial multiple coagulation factor deficiency	227300	AR	Sephardi and Oriental

Table 12.2. (continued)

Fragilitas oculi with joint hyperextensibility	229200	AR	Rare; Tunisian
German syndrome	231080	AR	3 of 4 affected families are Ashkenezi
Glanzmann thrombasthenia, Jewish type	273800.0001	AR	Sephardi
Glutathione peroxidase deficiency	138320	AD	Jews, unspecified
Glucose-6-phosphate dehydrogenase deficiency	305900	XLR	Sephardi / Oriental, esp. Kurdish
Glycogen storage disease III	232400	AR	Sephardi
Hyperbilirubinemia II / Dubin-Johnson syndrome	237500	AR	Iranian
Hyperbilirubinemia, transient neonatal familial	237900	AR	Yemenite
Ichthyosis vulgaris	146700	AD	India
Ichthyosis vulgaris	308100	XL	Iraq
Iminoglycinuria, type I	242600	AR	Ashkenazi
Iminoglycinuria, type II	138500	AD	Ashkenazi
Inclusion body myositis	147421	AD	2 cases in unrelated Iranian / Kurdish Jews
Infantile oplicatrophy with chorea and spastic paraplegia	258501	AR	Iraq
Keratosis palmoplantaris with peridontopathia and onychogryposis	245010	AR	"Cochin Jewish Disease"; India
Lactase deficiency	223100	AR	Jews, unspecified
Metachromatic leukodystrophy (late infantile type)	250100	AR	Habbanites (S. Arabia)
Mucopolysaccharidosis, type I (Hurler syndrome)	252800	AR	Decreased in Ashkenazi
Myasthenia, congenital with facial malformations	254195	AR	In 10 families of either Iraqi or Iranian Jews
Pachyonychia congenita	167200	AD	Jews, unspecified
Parotid salivary glycoprotein	168840	AD	Ashkenazi
Partial eosinophil peroxidase deficiency	261500	AR	Yemenite; of doubtful clinical significance

Table 12.2. (continued)

Disease	McKusick #	Probable or Known Pattern of Inheritance	Jewish Populations/ Comments
Pemphigus vulgaris	169610	AD	Jews, unspecified
Phenylketonuria	261600	AR	Sephardi/Oriental, esp. Yemenite; decreased in Ashkenazi
Pituatary dwarfism II (Larson type)	262500	AR	Sephardi/Oriental
Polycythemia vera		Non-Mendelian	Higher in Jewish than non-Jewish Americans
Polyglandular deficiency syndrome	263620	AR	All cases Persian Jews
Properdin deficiency	312060	XL	1 study with Sephardi of Tunisian origin
Pseudocholinesterase deficiency	177400	AD	Oriental (Iran/Iraq)
Pseudohypoaldosteronism, type I	264350	AR	Persian
Renal tubular acidosis with progressive nerve deafness	267300	AR	1 community in Kurdistan
Spondyloenchondrodysplasia	271550	AR	Apparent cases found in consanguineous Iraqi Jews
Susceptibility to hypervitaminosis A	240150	AR	European
Thalassemia (β)	141900	*AD, complex inheritance	Sephardi, esp. Kurdish
Usher syndrome	276900	AR	Jews in Berlin
Uric acid urolithiasis	191700	AD	Jews, unspecified
Werdnig Hoffman disease	253300	AR	Karaites
Wilson disease	277900	AR	Possible later onset and milder course in Jews (unspecified)
X-Linked properdin deficiency	312060	XLR	Sephardi Jews of Tunisian origin (1 Israeli study)

Sources: Mourant, Kopec, and Domaniewska-Sobczak (1978); Goodman (1979); McKusick (1994)
Note: AD, autosomal dominant; AR, autosomal recessive; XL, X-linked recessive

Judaism is a religion and culture of history and tradition. Its basic tenets are espoused in its stories and complex codified laws. Both of these constitute the traditional format against which many people measure their level of observance and/or cultural "Jewishness."

Most Jews believe that they are in some way descended not only traditionally but also biologically from those early Jews (Hebrews) identified in the Bible (the Torah [TOE-rah], also called the Five Books of Moses, and subsequent biblical texts), who arose from pastoral tribes inhabiting the mid-Euphrates valleys in the second millennium B.C.E.[2] The activities of these people are outlined clearly in the Bible dating from Abraham, identified as the first Jewish person, and extending through the story of the migrations of the Jews out of Egypt with Moses. With the departure from Egypt in the Exodus, the Jewish people returned to their ancient homeland in the area of modern-day Israel and founded the first Jewish state. This is chronicled through other books in the Bible marking the rise of the rule by kings, the building and destruction of two great temples, and the eventual dispersion of the Jewish people throughout the Near East and ancient world by a variety of foreign powers. A number of Jewish holidays and religious ceremonies mark the incidents of this ancient history[3] (Sachar, 1967).

During these centuries of dispersal, or "Diaspora," Jewish history becomes more nebulous. A variety of centers of Jewish life developed, particularly throughout much of Europe, extending outward around the world. These are presumed to derive from the continued integrity of the early dispersed populations and have persisted in their present geographical locations for centuries. Many contemporary Jews who have emigrated (primarily to the Western Hemisphere and Israel) retain a strong sense of their recent geographical and cultural background. As with other immigrant populations, first-generation Jewish immigrants retain the language of their country of origin.

DEMOGRAPHICS

Given the difficulties in identifying who is Jewish beyond self-report, estimation of the size of Jewish populations is difficult. General estimates in the last decade place the current world Jewish population at around 14 million, with approximately 7 million living in the United States, 4 million in Israel, and 3 million scattered elsewhere in the world. The latter include large enclaves in the former Soviet Union as well as substantial populations in South America, Western Europe, North Africa, and the Middle East outside Israel. Smaller populations exist in the Indian subcontinent and Asia (Beaver, 1982).

Estimates of the level of observance in these populations are even more difficult, though large percentages of secular and Reform Jews can be found in the United States. In a recent survey, approximately 7 million adults in the United States (2.7% of the U.S. population) identify themselves as either Jewish or of Jewish background. About 5.5 million consider themselves observant in some manner. The denominational distribution is: 38 percent Reform, 35.1 percent Conservative, 19.5 percent "just Jewish" or "something else," 6.1 percent Orthodox, and 1.3 percent Reconstructionist (Goldstein, 1992).

ASHKENAZIC AND SEPHARDIC JEWS

Two large general groups are conventionally considered to constitute the bulk of the Jewish population: Ashkenazi [ASH-ken-AH-zee], those who identify themselves as Northern or Eastern European in origin; and Sephardi [sef-AHRD-dee], those who are of Mediterranean or Iberian origin.[4] Ashkenazic Jews (or *Ashkenazim*) share a variety of religious and linguistic traditions, developed over centuries in Poland, Germany, the Balkans, eastern Russia, Estonia, Lithuania, and Latvia, and elsewhere in Eastern Europe. Their religious traditions are based on the growth of great rabbinic schools scattered throughout these areas in the Middle Ages. Their interpretations of the Bible and the Talmud [TAL-moud], the compendium of religious law developed over some thousand years beginning around B.C.E. 500, were codified by the middle of the sixteenth century into a comprehensive set of rules delineating the moral and legal responsibilities of the observant Jew. All activities from the time of awakening to going to sleep are covered explicitly for both men and women. To this day, the most observant Jews (Orthodox) attempt to follow this "way of life" as much as possible.

The Ashkenazic Jewish tradition may be most familiar to Americans, since the majority of Jews in the United States currently are of Ashkenazi background. This tradition is familiar in the works of such writers as Sholom Alechem, Chaim Potok, and Philip Roth and cinematographers like

Woody Allen. Ashkenazim are linguistically linked through Yiddish [YID-ish], essentially a form of Middle German written with Hebrew characters, which became the common language in use throughout European Jewish culture. With Hebrew as the formal religious language, as well as the official language of the modern State of Israel, the use of Yiddish has decreased dramatically in the United States, though it remains a common language for many Jews worldwide.

Sephardic Jews have a comparably rich history and tradition. This group has its origins in Moorish Spain and other cultural and religious centers. With the expulsion of the Jews from Spain in 1492 and the subsequent Spanish Diaspora, Jewish populations from this region spread throughout the Old World (along the shores of the Mediterranean, with large cultural centers in Turkey) as well as to the New World. The Sephardim were the major founders of the first Jewish communities in both North and South America and formed the majority of the New World's Jewish population for the first several hundred years of the European immigration. Not until the great emigrations from Eastern Europe in this century did the Ashkenazic Jews become the predominant Jewish community in the Americas. Like Ashkenazic Jews, Sephardic Jews are also linked by a common language, known as Ladino [la-DEE-no].

Jews typically speak the major language of their country, so with the exception of first-generation immigrants, language should not be a significant problem in genetic counseling.

LEVELS OF ORTHODOXY

An important dimension in any of these geographic or ethnic groups is what might be considered the level of orthodoxy or adherence to traditional practices and interpretation of Jewish law. It is not likely that any categorical scheme will please all Jewish individuals. Most who identify themselves as practicing or observant Jews perceive their observance of Jewish law to be appropriate. One dichotomy that has been proposed is between "Halakic" [hal-AH-kik] Jews (from the Hebrew word meaning "established Jewish law") and what might be termed "non-Halakic" Jews (i.e., those who see the law as divinely inspired but more open to interpretation). However, there is a conventionally recognized spectrum of orthodoxy based on the role that religious life and tenets play in determining the details of daily life.

On the most basic level, one might divide the Jewish community into three groups: those who practice Orthodox Judaism in one of several forms; observant but less-orthodox Jews; and "secular" Jews, who identify themselves as Jewish by heritage but are not particularly observant.

Orthodox and Ultra-Orthodox

Although many Orthodox Jews are indistinguishable by dress or habit in the secular world, their religious practice and outlook on their lives are much more informed by the dictates of traditional religious law and guidelines. Religious worship and daily activities are more clearly prescribed. For example, since vehicular travel, which represents work, is prohibited on the Sabbath, Orthodox Jews will often live close to their houses of worship. On the Sabbath, they walk to religious services.

Considerably distinct from other denominations are groupings of Jews who are called Ultra-Orthodox. Individuals who identify with this level of religious observance are most likely to have alterations in hairstyle and / or dress, related to strict observance of interpretations of Jewish law and custom. Men frequently dress in black, with fringes of fabric visible at the belt line. Their heads are almost always covered with either a *kippah* [KEY-paw] or *yarmulke* [YAH-muck-uh]. Married women in the Ultra-Orthodox community frequently shear their hair very short and wear a wig (known in Yiddish as a *shaytl* [SHAY-til]). Women cover their heads in the presence of men other than their husbands.

Stereotypical roles for men and women are well defined in Ultra-Orthodox communities. Men often make final decisions and occupy themselves with religious obligations and providing a livelihood. Women typically follow the dictates of their husbands, brothers, or fathers and attend to prescribed activities concerned with bearing and raising children.

Women and men are frequently separated, and contact between the sexes, except in marriage, is strictly curtailed. Accordingly, it would be inappropriate for a female genetic counselor to touch an Ultra-Orthodox male, even to shake hands or to offer comfort; likewise, for a male genetic counselor to touch a woman, either married or unmarried. Similarly, issues may arise regarding physical examination of patients of the opposite sex, and the physician may need to discuss procedures and gain approval before proceeding.

The most commonly identified Ultra-Orthodox groups are collectively known as Hasidim. Members of this denomination trace their philosophic origins back to seventeenth-century Poland. The movement subsequently splintered into a variety of sects, often headed by charismatic religious leaders, rebbes [REB-bays]. The best known of these sects is the Lubavitcher Hasids.

Ultra-Orthodox Jews generally live in enclaves within cities, the majority of which center around the eastern seaboard of the United States and in Israel. In Ultra-Orthodox communities, adherence to tradition and religious laws necessitates dialogue and explanation in terms of genetic counseling. Strict adherence to religious obligations—holidays beginning in the evening, keeping of the Sabbath from Friday evening to Saturday evening, various obligatory fast days, dietary observances, lack of physical contact between unmarried men and women, traditional roles for men and women, and general prohibitions against abortion and autopsy—presents areas with which those doing genetic counseling should at least be familiar. Teams of rabbis have spent years reviewing the impact of specific new technologies (in vitro fertilization, prenatal testing) and their impact on the breadth and intent of Jewish law. Some familiarity with the religious orientations toward these major issues in the community being served, therefore, is useful, and consultation with the individual's rabbis may be not only helpful but necessary.

Reform, Conservative, and Reconstructionist

Those Jews who are affiliated with a particular level of orthodoxy but are not considered Orthodox include, in the three largest groupings, Reform, Conservative, and Reconstructionist. The Reform movement developed during the latter part of the nineteenth century in reaction to the orthodoxy of most Jewish practice in the Ashkenazi world. In Reform Judaism, religious law is not viewed as divinely revealed or binding (Kolatch, 1981, 1985). Liberalization and adaptation to the surrounding culture and the removal of many formal and traditional religious activities were hallmarks of the Reform movement's origins.

Conservative Judaism developed in reaction to the liberalism of the Reform movement, with a return to some more traditional modes of worship. Conservative Jews consider the Torah to have been revealed by God, thus authoritative and immutable, but leave more room for interpretation than the most orthodox.

The Reconstructionist movement is the youngest denomination. It attempts to reinterpret the orthodox intent of Jewish law in the light of modern day. Reconstructionism has been described as a "middle road" between Reform and Conservative Judaism, its tenets being that one can be a practicing Jew in a variety of ways (Kolatch, 1981, 1985).

A strong feminist movement is also emerging, especially in the more liberal portions of Judaism. It seeks to remove some of the traditional patriarchy from Judaism and enlarge the scope of roles for women.

Secular

"Secular" Jews may come from any background of Jewish religious life. The unifying principle of this group is that they practice religion on a very personal basis, often outside of formal religious acts or ceremonies. These individuals are usually "unaffiliated," that is, not associated with a specific congregation, synagogue, or temple.

One major difference between affiliated and unaffiliated (including, but not limited to, secular) Jews is an association with a rabbi, who might be best described as a religious organizer in their lives. Many non-Jews consider rabbis to be the equivalent of priests or ministers. However, rabbis are generally more independent in terms of their religious interpretations and are more accurately considered interpreters and arbiters of Jewish law. Accordingly, they serve more as teachers for their congregation than as mediators of individuals' religious lives. Rabbis are trained within each of the major religious groupings in Judaism. Their training includes interpretation of Jewish law as well as organization of congregations and religious instruction.

IMPLICATIONS FOR GENETIC SERVICES

As we have stated, many Jews identify with specific denominations within Jewish culture. Judaism, however, emphasizes individual religious observance. In addition, when dealing with issues often addressed in genetic counseling, individuals' attitudes and decisions may be affected in surprising ways both by memories of how parents or grandparents may have dealt with similar issues and by consultation with more traditional sources, such as rabbis or more orthodox friends or family members (Steiner-Grossman and David, 1993).

It should be recognized that the identification of an individual's affiliation and / or cultural and geographic background, while useful as a starting point, cannot substitute for a thorough exploration of the individual's perspective. Also, recourse to religious support or guidance may be needed at any point with any specific individual or family.

Holidays and the Jewish Calendar

Jewish culture celebrates a number of major holidays each year. With the exception of the High Holidays—Rosh Hashana [ROSH ha-SHAH-nah] (the New Year) and Yom Kippur [YAWM-kee-POOR] (the Day of Atonement)—all are related to historical events. Jewish tradition follows a lunar calendar 354 days long. To harmonize with the Gregorian calendar, extra months and / or days are added according to a complicated schedule (leap years occur seven times every nineteen years). For this reason, Jewish holidays occur at different times in the Gregorian calendar from year to year. The day (and therefore the beginning of a holiday or the Sabbath) officially begins and ends at sundown.

Depending on the level of orthodoxy and personal practice, holidays may be of significance and need to be taken into account when scheduling individuals for genetic counseling or other medical activities. For example, almost all observant Jews believe Yom Kippur, one of the holiest days in the year, to be a day requiring obligatory religious activity. Observant Jews will cease everyday work-related activities relatively early in the afternoon to go home and prepare for the onset of this holiday, which includes prayer and fasting. Almost all practicing Jews would probably resist any attempt to arrange for anything but the most necessary surgery on this day. While Yom Kippur is celebrated once a year, many observant Jews consider the Sabbath just as holy, though it occurs on a weekly basis. Taking these traditions into account when appointments and other activities are scheduled will lessen inconvenience and possibly compliance problems.

Illness and Medicine

Judaism has a strong historical or traditional set of mystical beliefs. These reflect ancient cultural interpretations of major life changes such as birth and death. However, a direct relationship between maternal experience during pregnancy (beyond routine medical considerations) and pregnancy outcome is not typically perceived in Jewish tradition. Regardless, Jewish individuals throughout the world, particularly those where science holds less sway, will frequently have belief systems about appropriate and risky behavior during pregnancy. This occurs with newborns, as well. Traditionally, observers are loath to overzealously compliment a newborn infant to avoid invoking the jealousy of evil powers. In addition, a variety of observances occur around death or burial, related to traditional beliefs about activities of spirits, including those of the deceased.

There are no strong mystical traditions about genetic disorders. In Judaism, illness is generally seen as amenable to human intervention along with divine intervention, rather than exclusively one or the other. Most individuals who would identify themselves as outside the Ultra-Orthodox community have what might be termed a naturalistic or scientific view of health and illness as originating in the physical world and the body rather than in the spiritual world.

Judaism also has a long tradition of respect for medicine and health professions. There is, therefore, no primary conflict between Jewish religious belief and general medical practices. The preservation of health and support for the activities of medicine are accorded priority in religious law through an overriding tradition known as Pikuach Nefesh [peh-KOO-akch NEH-fesh] ("saving" or "prolonging life"), which some scholars identify as among the most basic principles of Jewish law (Kolatch, 1985). According to this concept, prescribed rituals (e.g., fasting, circumcision) may be deferred or foregone if participation presents a risk to life or health. A long tradition of stories and interpretations is associated with this concept. The concept of Pikuach Nefesh has been invoked in support of such modern technologies as organ transplantation. Indeed, the provision of medical assistance is recognized as desirable, or even an obligation.

Marriage, Conception, and Pregnancy

Arranged marriages, facilitated by marriage brokers, have been a familiar feature of Jewish culture until recent times. In some current Orthodox and Ultra-Orthodox communities, marriages are still arranged or decisions regarding marriage strongly influenced by the opinions of important authorities in the family.

Jewish tradition places strong emphasis on procreation as the natural outcome of marriage. While the majority of Jews have personally informed opinions about the termination of pregnancy, this choice is generally in disfavor in the Orthodox and Ultra-Orthodox communities according to interpretations of Jewish law. Thus, the modern understanding of genetic, particularly autosomal recessive, conditions and those known to exist more frequently in certain Jewish populations (e.g., Tay Sachs disease, Gaucher disease, and various haplotypes of cystic fibrosis; see table 12.1) presents difficult dilemmas for Orthodox and Ultra-Orthodox Jews. An awareness of this situation is of obvious importance in genetic counseling with more orthodox Jews. Divorce, it might be noted, while not taken lightly, is permitted under Jewish law.

The Orthodox community in the greater New York City area has developed an ingenious mechanism through an organization known as Dor Yeshorim [DOOR yeh-SHOR-im] for decreasing the need for either prenatal testing or the termination of pregnancy for fetuses affected with the more familiar conditions (Lefkowitz, 1992). Individuals wishing to arrange marriages either for themselves or for their children submit blood samples for haplotype testing. Evaluations are done through Dor Yeshorim to identify carriers in this population. These individuals are not publicly identified, but marriages in which both partners will be carriers of specific recessive conditions can be identified. Couples who are contemplating marriage can then contact Dor Yeshorim with their identifying number to learn if their match is "compatible" from a genetic point of view. Accordingly, without individuals or even other family members being informed of their carrier status, marriages can be arranged that have much lower risks of producing affected children. This maintains individual privacy and permits the continuation of a traditional method of entering into marriage, yet avoids the expected high frequency of children affected with specific conditions. It utilizes neither pregnancy termination nor unusual methods of conception (GIFT, in vitro fertilization, or artificial insemination by a donor) to maintain continuity within the community.

Outside of the Orthodox community, marriages are almost never arranged and genetic counselors will be faced with classic genetic counseling issues. Individuals of specific known ethnic backgrounds will require consultation and sometimes, if possible, preconceptional and / or prenatal testing for couples who are thought to be at risk. This has been the case for a number of years with respect to Tay Sachs disease and other conditions, and these considerations will be familiar to most genetic counselors.

A further comment on technologically dependent conception is in order. The use of artificial insemination by a donor or GIFT requires the provision of sperm or eggs from someone not involved in either the marriage or the relationship. However, Jewishness is matrilineally defined, with the children's religion determined by the mother's religion. Accordingly, a child born to a Jewish woman where artificial insemination by a donor is used would not require the identification of the sperm as coming from a Jewish male. However, a child conceived via GIFT might need to undergo formal conversion to be considered Jewish if the religion of the woman who donated the egg is unknown or not Jewish. Reform Jews have expanded their definition of Jewishness to include the religion of the father; thus, formal conversion would not be an issue.

While intermarriage (marriage with someone outside of the Jewish faith) is frowned on in every denomination of Judaism, it is relatively common outside of the Orthodox community. It is worth reiterating in this regard that cultural issues of Judaism pertain to people who identify themselves as Jewish or who continue to practice traditions that they perceive as occurring in their family. However, genetic risks are limited to those who are descended from the large regional Jewish populations or who might be termed ethnically Jewish. Individuals who have been raised outside of Judaism may still have grandparents who were Jewish and from populations known to be at risk, and therefore need counseling about genetic disorders found in those ethnic groups. Similarly, individuals may convert to Judaism and require culturally sensitive genetic counseling for their particular beliefs but not face the carrier status issues that are found in ethnic Jews. When taking a family history, the genetic counselor should identify both the ethnic origin and the cultural orientation before proceeding with counseling.

Orthodox Jewish traditions followed by some groups may prescribe the frequency and timing of conjugal relations between husband and wife. This is not a significant issue in general genetic counseling, but fertility counselors working with Orthodox couples should be aware of issues such as proscriptions against sexual contact between husband and wife around the time of menses, during fast days, and in times of mourning. An additional note with regard to sexuality is that the Orthodox community does not look on contraception with favor. These practices and attitudes are generally not issues among Jews of less orthodox denominations and merit less consideration with these individuals.

Although Judaism recognizes procreation as a principal element of the divine plan, issues regarding appropriate behavior during pregnancy are related primarily to an individual's cultural background rather than religious doctrine. Thus, an exploration of cultural attitudes toward pregnancy with individual couples is in order. However, the knowledge that someone is Jewish or of a particular local culture does not suggest what the important issues might be for that individual.

Birth and Rites of Passage

Birth is an event surrounded by a number of Jewish rituals, many of which are retained even by secular Jews. Traditionally, birth is conceptualized as occurring at the time the baby's head "crowns" (i.e., when the head is visible and delivery is usually able to proceed). Judaism, therefore, differs significantly from Christian, especially Catholic, determination in this area. Until this point in the birth process, the Jewish infant is not considered to be a separate, independent life. Before crowning, therefore, if a decision between the survival of the mother and the infant is necessary, the mother, who has the potential to have other children, is selected rather than the infant (Jakobovits, 1975). This is an area about which most Jews themselves (except the most orthodox) are unfamiliar. Exploration of this area will be important if questions arise about the management of a pregnancy or subsequent deliveries specifically related to genetic conditions that might make vaginal birth difficult.

One of the basic tenets of Judaic tradition is that all male Jews be circumcised. The customary date for circumcision is the eighth day of life. The circumcision ceremony, generally known as a bris (var. brith), is traditionally performed in the family's home by a *mohel* [MOI-yel], an individual trained in the ritual of circumcision. The procedure marks the admission of the male child into Jewish tradition. Circumcision can be deferred for a variety of reasons, such as abnormalities in the formation of the urethra, the need for surgery, or potential health risk. Similarly, an infant born prematurely does not have to be circumcised eight days after his delivery, but the ceremony would be expected eight days after he is out of danger. The circumcision itself, rather than the ritual, is the primary requirement. The participation of a mohel, though traditional, is not required. Thus, many Jewish infants are circumcised in the hospital by physicians without a religious ceremony. However, when this is done, an additional ceremony is required to sanction the religious meaning of the circumcision.

An additional ritual associated with male infants known as Pidyan Haben [PID-yahn ha-BEN] is more rarely performed, though it may be utilized by Jews of any denomination. In a tradition that dates back to biblical times, the first-born males of all manners of animals and humans were dedicated to the service or control of the priests in the original temple of Solomon. The ritual symbolically acknowledges this, in that the first-born male child delivered vaginally is "subject" to this tradition. Generally at thirty days after birth (or thirty days after health and stability are attained), the family of the first-born male infant may celebrate this tradition. Infants delivered by nonvaginal methods are not eligible, nor are subsequent sons if the woman has had a prior miscarriage, even if it is the first-born male. The ceremony is performed only on living healthy children, so the loss of a stillborn male or the loss of products of conception alter a family's "eligibility" to celebrate this tradition. No data are available on how commonly this ritual is currently celebrated, though it may play a significant enough role to affect the functioning of certain families. The loss of a first-born male child before this ceremony or difficulty in participation due to other problems such as genetic conditions may merit exploration in genetic counseling.

Among the more orthodox Jews, the birth of a girl has been celebrated with joy but without particular traditional markers or ceremonies, with the exception of naming at a subsequent service in the temple. The dearth of ritual accompanying female birth may reflect, in part, a tendency in Jewish communities of a century or more ago to emphasize the importance of the birth of sons, or at least one son. This is not to say that any particular couple would prefer a child of one sex or another, nor do Jews practice prenatal sex selection for male children. But in some more traditional families, subtle pressures to produce sons may exist. In addition, the birth of a son with a genetic condition that would not permit the continuation of the family line might raise special distressing issues (though the birth of any child with difficulties is distressing in any family).

In some Conservative and in almost all Reform temples, a separate tradition of naming a female child approximately thirty days after birth has developed. Boys are traditionally named formally at the time of circumcision. As in many cultures, names are considered to have particular power and importance. In Ashkenazic tradition, the names of the living are not used to name children, so it would be unusual for traditional Jewish families to call children "Junior." They do believe, however, that it is important to keep names alive. The names of children who died young are not used again in the same nuclear family, but the names of ancestors are frequently used to honor both the memory and the child. Girls and boys are frequently given Hebrew names (in addition to names in the family's first language), which are not routinely used in less orthodox communities. Another Ashkenazic tradition followed occasionally is the renaming of children (or adults) facing a life-threatening illness. The purpose of this is to confuse the Angel of Death, who approaches looking for a particular person.

Naming is also important in Sephardic tradition, where frequently names are continued through families. Sephardic Jews may utilize names of the living as well as those of deceased ancestors. Therefore, for many Jews, especially for many Orthodox families, the discovery that a child has a genetic condition that may shorten life or impair fertility may have ramifications not only for the family directly but also for the loss of a name, which may have been chosen to honor a dear family member or friend.

Rites of passage in Judaism are better known throughout Western culture than they were a century or two ago. The ritual initiation into adult responsibilities occurs for males (bar mitzvah [BAR MITZ-vah]) around the age of thirteen. The age is not a matter of rigid rule; the ceremony can occur at any time when an individual is considered to have the necessary maturity and ability to perform the ceremonies in the denomination. Many practicing Jews, usually not Ultra-Orthodox, also celebrate an initiation into adulthood for females (bat mitzvah). Marriage, as noted, is also a major cultural expectation for Jews. Awareness of these transitional traditions is of obvious importance in counseling families with children whose genetic conditions may affect their cognitive and physical development and abilities.

In addition, with regard to mental retardation, Judaism has always recognized differences in abilities and adjusts expectations accordingly. Birth defects raise more complex issues, but life is generally valued over nonlife.

Death

Respect for the dead is a major Judaic principle. The practices which surround death and its commemoration are of importance to those counseling families with a potential genetic diagnosis. Jewish tradition avoids open coffins and espouses the idea of rapid burial as long as most family members can arrive in time. It is Jewish tradition, but not law, that individuals be buried generally within a day or two of their death. By tradition, funerals involve plain pine caskets. A variety of rules surround funerals and burial. For the Orthodox, the body of the deceased is never left alone between the moment of death and interment, and Orthodox participants will pray around the body of the deceased.

The requirements of respect for the dead and rapid burial have raised a difficult set of problems for traditional Judaism with regard to autopsy. Autopsy, in fact, has been routinely discouraged, if not banned outright. However, in keeping with the concept of Pikuach Nefesh ("saving life"), the fact that an autopsy might provide information of benefit to the living is a powerful recommendation for its authorization. It is wise to involve religious counseling when giving genetic counseling to anyone who identifies this as an area of difficulty. A rabbinic decision may be required to determine whether or not an autopsy may be performed.

In the context of ceremonies associated with death and burial, it is worth noting an additional categorization of Jews. Practicing Jews are grouped into three major categories: those who identify themselves as descended from priests ("Kohayn" [KO-HAYN]), those descended from assistants ("Levites" [LEE-vites]), and the remainder of the Jewish people ("Yisroel" [YIS-ro-ail]). Many less-orthodox Jews are unaware of the grouping to which they belong, but among the Orthodox there are prohibitions against the "Kohayn" coming in contact with anything considered unclean, including cemeteries and the dead. It is not uncommon, therefore, for Orthodox practitioners not to be able to attend the funerals of even family members, due to their membership in this "hereditary" (patrilinear) group.

The death of the close family member, particularly a first-degree relative, requires participation in a variety of mourning rituals. For more observant Jews there are a series of progressively less restricted time periods requiring abstinence from participation in activities of daily life. Many Jews and non-Jews are familiar with the period of *shiva [SHIH-vah]* (meaning "seven," the obligatory number of days of mourning), where first-degree relatives gather in a home to mourn the passing of an individual. In Ashkenazic tradition, mirrors are covered. A variety of explanations are given: to avoid vanity, to avoid further distress by seeing one's own grief, to avoid letting the spirit of the dead person see itself.

In Jewish tradition, mourners wear either torn ribbons or torn clothing to represent their grief. During the mourning period they sit on wooden stools or chairs lower than those around them, a practice known as "sitting shiva." Religious ceremonies are held in the home each day and individuals refrain from normal activities, even cooking. Accordingly, friends and neighbors frequently bring meals and food for both the mourners and visitors. In Jewish tradition, food, rather than flowers, is given during periods of mourning. More Orthodox Jews refrain from many public activities for the first month and some for the first year after the death of a close family member. Observant Jews go to the synagogue each morning for approximately a year to offer the Kaddish (KAH-dish ["Mourner's Prayer for the Dead"]).

Anniversaries of a death are commemorated by the lighting of a Yahrzeit (YAR-tsite) candle. Since Judaism follows a lunar rather than an adapted solar calendar, the anniversaries of a death may vary markedly on the Gregorian calendar from year to year. Since those involved in genetic counseling are often sensitive to the difficulties that "anniversary" presents, special attention may be required to discover whether or not a family is in fact aware of and addressing these sorts of issues.

The Jewish tradition places little emphasis on an afterlife, although there is a belief in an immortal soul. Orthodox Jews believe in the resurrection of the body with the arrival of the Messiah, but concepts of heaven and hell are not central to Jewish tradition. While these concepts exist, punishments during afterlife are not major motivations for the observance of Jewish law. The concepts of purgatory and limbo are alien to Jewish tradition. Suicide is considered a serious offense in Jewish law; thus, suicides are excluded from burial in Jewish cemeteries, and obtaining information about this as a cause of death may be problematic, especially with more orthodox Jews.

Genetic Diseases

The conditions listed in tables 12.1 and 12.2 have been reported (or appear) to occur with increased frequency in various Jewish populations. Since many of these populations represent groups that have been isolated for generations and for whom intermarriage was or is common, the presence of rare, apparently autosomal recessive conditions is not surprising. Conditions for which only one familial occurrence is reported, or that are not clearly increased in a Jewish population, have not been included. Readers are referred to the comprehensive works by Goodman (1979) and Mourant, Kopec, and Domaniewska-Sobczak (1978), as well as McKusick (1994).

CONCLUSION

It is difficult even within Judaism to reach consensus on the meaning or importance of practices within the various levels of orthodoxy. Accordingly, this chapter should be viewed as merely an introduction, one perspective on a complex subject. Readers are encouraged to consult more detailed discussions, both specific to genetics (especially Goodman, 1979; Mourant, Kopec, and Domaniewska-Sobczak, 1978; and Bonne-Tamir and Adam, 1992) and concerning practice and culture in general (e.g., Kolatch, 1981, 1985).

SUMMARY

—Ascertain the level of observance of Judaism from the family before beginning any counseling session.
—Do not schedule clinics for Friday evening or Saturday. Also, be aware that many Jewish holidays are not marked on most calendars. Simply ask when scheduling appointments.

—GIFT or in vitro fertilization may be viewed as an unusual method of conception and may not be acceptable if the egg donor is not Jewish.

—Among more orthodox Jews, artificial insemination by a donor may be considered acceptable because a child's religion is determined matrilineally. Among some Jews, artificial insemination by a donor is an option only if the donor is not Jewish, thereby decreasing the risk of consanguinity.

—Autopsy is generally discouraged, unless there is a powerful recommendation for it. Discussion and advice from a rabbi may be needed.

—The utilization of prenatal diagnosis will vary widely, depending on the cultural and religious orientation.

—In Orthodox families, the male is often the decision maker, but may need to consult a rabbi. Try to schedule prenatal testing early enough in a pregnancy to allow time for such consultation in the event that issues do arise.

—Orthodox families will probably have their own internal support groups, while less-observant Jews may utilize support groups outside their immediate community.

—Members of smaller, isolated Jewish enclaves may have a higher probability of consanguinity, raising the likelihood that rare, or "private," recessive syndromes may appear.

ACKNOWLEDGMENTS

We thank Rabbi Jeffrey Bennett for his consultation and critical review of the manuscript, as well as Kathleen Faniel for her transcription services.

NOTES

1. Traditionally, an individual is Jewish whose biological mother is Jewish or who has converted according to prescribed rituals. By legal statute in the modern State of Israel, individuals who fulfill these criteria are entitled to immigrate and receive Israeli citizenship.

2. Common usage in the West has included the time notations B.C. ("before Christ") and A.D. ("Anno Domini," "in the year of our Lord"). Since these terms have religious connotations, it is standard practice among many observant Jews to use the alternatives B.C.E. ("before the common era") for B.C. and C.E. ("common era") for A.D.

3. This biblical history forms the basis of almost all Jewish traditions, with some exceptions. Noteworthy among these would be the Ethiopian Jewish population, known as Falashas, who date their conversion from the time of Solomon and the Queen of Sheba. They are an ancient Jewish population who share many early religious texts but for whom the majority of elaborated laws and interpretations of early texts are not part of the cultural tradition. Most of the remaining Falashas have migrated to Israel, where attempts are being made to incorporate them into modern Israeli society.

4. In their monograph primarily on blood grouping of Jews, Mourant et al. (1978)

devoted separate chapters to Jews of Palestine, Samaritans, Oriental Jews, Yemenite Jews, Karaites, Jews of Africa, as well as Sephardic and Ashkenazic Jews.

REFERENCES

Beaver, R. P., et al. 1982. *Eerdman's Handbook to the World's Religions.* Herts, U.K.: Lion Publishing.

Bonne-Tamir, B., and Adam, A. 1992. *Genetic Diversity among Jews: Diseases and Markers at the DNA Level.* New York: Oxford University Press.

Feldman, D. M. 1986. The ethical implications of new reproductive technologies. In Meier, L. (ed.), *Jewish Values in Bioethics,* pp. 174–82. New York: Human Sciences Press.

Goldstein, S. 1992. Profile of American jewry: Insights from the 1990 National Jewish Population Survey. In Singer, D., and Seldon, R. R. (eds.), *American Jewish Yearbook, 1992,* pp. 76–173. New York: American Jewish Committee.

Goodman, R. M. 1979. *Genetic Disorders among the Jewish People.* Baltimore: Johns Hopkins University Press.

Jakobovits, I. 1975. *Jewish Medical Ethics.* New York: Bloch Publishing.

Kolatch, A. J. 1981. *The Jewish Book of Why.* Middle Village, N.Y.: Jonathan David Publishers.

———. 1985. *The Second Jewish Book of Why.* Middle Village, N.Y.: Jonathan David Publishers.

Lefkowitz, S. 1992. Dor Yeshorim: A grass roots success story. *Genesis: The Newsletter of the Genetics Network of the Empire State* 4:1–2.

McKusick, V. A. 1994. *Mendelian Inheritance in Man: Catalogs of Autosomal Dominant, Autosomal Recessive, and X-Linked Phenotypes.* 11th ed. Baltimore: Johns Hopkins University Press.

Mourant, A. E., Kopec, A. C., and Domaniewska-Sobczak, K. 1978. *The Genetics of the Jews.* Oxford: Clarendon Press.

Sachar, A. L. 1967. *A History of the Jews.* New York: Alfred A. Knopf.

Steiner-Grossman, P., and David, K. L. 1993. Involvement of rabbis in counseling and referral for genetic conditions: Results of a survey. *American Journal of Human Genetics* 53:1359–65.

13

Deaf Culture

Jamie Israel, M.S.,
Margaret Cunningham, R.N.,
Helen Thumann, M.A., and
Kathleen Shaver Arnos, Ph.D.

Almost 21 million Americans are reported to have some type of hearing loss, which may range from mild to profound (Hotchkiss, 1989). Deafness is heterogeneous, having many genetic and environmental causes. Genetic types of deafness may be congenital or may develop in childhood or adulthood. To date, over four hundred different forms of genetic hearing loss have been described; approximately one-third of these occur as part of a complex syndrome. These types can be distinguished by the pattern of inheritance, audiologic characteristics, age at onset, and clinical course (Konigsmark and Gorlin, 1976; Gorlin, Toriello, and Cohen, 1995).

The incidence of congenital severe to profound deafness in the United States is approximately one in one thousand births, representing between two thousand and four thousand infants born each year (Bergstrom, 1980). Complex segregation analysis has been used to determine that at least 50 percent of these cases have a genetic etiology, with approximately 60 to 80 percent inherited in an autosomal recessive mode, 15 to 30 percent in a dominant mode, and 1 to 2 percent X-linked (Fraser, 1976; Rose, Conneally, and

---

In this chapter, the term *deaf* is used to denote a person who audiologically has a hearing loss that may range from mild to profound and may be sensorineural, conductive, or mixed. The term *Deaf* is used to denote cultural deafness.

Nance, 1977). Recent DNA linkage technology has been applied to the localization of genes for various types of hereditary deafness (Barker et al., 1990; Foy et al., 1990; Lewis et al., 1990; Kumar et al., 1994; Kimberling et al., 1995). This technology has great potential for increasing our understanding of the specific genes involved.

Health care providers have had little exposure to the cultural, linguistic, and communication factors that may present barriers when deaf people attempt to gain access to medical services and receive good quality health care (DiPietro, Knight, and Sams, 1981). Recently, awareness has increased about large segments of the U.S. population, including deaf people, being medically underserved due to linguistic, cultural, and religious differences, geographic isolation, and/or poverty (Biesecker, Magyari, and Paul, 1987; Paul and Kavanagh, 1990). More attention has been given to the special communication needs of deaf adults in the medical setting (Davenport, 1977; Langham-Brown, 1981; DiPietro and Knight, 1982; Wood, 1987; McEwen and Anton-Culver, 1988; Meyers, Melhado, and Frances, 1989), as well as to issues specific to genetic counseling (Boughman and Shaver, 1982; Israel, 1989; Arnos, 1990). These recent efforts may help reduce barriers and increase access to medical services.

Deaf individuals are part of a minority group based on their audiologic commonalities. However, deaf people are also individuals whose cultural beliefs, language, and modes of communication may vary. This chapter addresses some of the cultural, linguistic, and communication differences that exist in the deaf population, some of the potential barriers to access and use of medical and genetic counseling services, and methods that may increase good quality genetic services for this population.

LANGUAGE ACQUISITION

Many factors contribute to a deaf person's communication preferences and abilities and the acquisition of English (manual, verbal, and/or written) or American Sign Language (ASL). For example, the age at onset of hearing loss may be a significant factor. The deafness can occur at or close to the time of birth or develop after the acquisition of a verbal language. Additionally, the degree of the hearing loss and the benefit of hearing aids and/or use of residual hearing may be contributing factors. Whether parents or family members are deaf or hearing, their primary language, and how the family communicates may also significantly affect a young child's acquisition of language and subsequent educational and communication choices.

In the United States, approximately 90 percent of deaf individuals come from families in which both parents have normal hearing (Rawlings and Jensema, 1977); the primary mode of communication in the home is spoken English. For these hearing parents, the diagnosis of deafness in their child may be their first exposure to deafness. They may be uncertain about the choices they must begin to make about their child's education, and how the child and family will communicate.

Language acquisition for a hearing child of hearing parents begins in infancy and occurs through the continuous exposure to language that is heard through interaction with or being around others (including family, peers, and neighbors) and through contact with television and radio (DiPietro, Knight, and Sams, 1981; DiPietro and Knight, 1982). Many deaf children whose parents are hearing may not have these opportunities for acquiring language, communication, and learning about the world. As a result, when a deaf child of hearing parents enters elementary school, he or she often lags behind children with normal hearing in the areas of language skills (spoken English or sign language), general knowledge about the world, and social adaptability. Many of the 10 percent of deaf children who are born to deaf families acquire the natural language used by their deaf parents (American Sign Language) and have a greater knowledge base about themselves, their family, and the world around them (Johnson, Liddell, and Erting, 1989; Meadow-Orlans, 1990).

Formal education also has a profound influence on the acquisition and refinement of language. The type of school attended, the communication mode used, and the interaction with other deaf peers and adults in the school and home environment all contribute to a deaf person's acquisition of spoken, written, and / or manual language. Educational options may include residential schools for deaf children, day-school programs for deaf students, self-contained day classes through public school systems, and mainstreamed classes where deaf children attend class with hearing classmates for all or parts of the day (National Information Center on Deafness, 1987b). The communication focus of these educational settings may differ: some programs use one system or a combination of sign language systems (ASL and / or English), and some use speechreading and speech exclusively (oral communication); other programs adopt a philosophy of total communication which accepts and uses a range of communication modes, including sign, spoken English, and speechreading.

Deaf education during the last two centuries has faced much conflict and debate over how deaf students should communicate and how, where, and what they should be taught (Moores, 1990). Although educational opportunities for deaf individuals have increased, many researchers believe that our educational system has failed to meet the needs of deaf students (Johnson, Liddell, and Erting, 1989). Studies of school achievement have shown that deaf students continue to fall behind hearing children throughout their school years. In 1983, the scaled score performances on the reading comprehension and the mathematics computation subtests of the Stanford Achievement Test were measured for deaf high school students. The mean reading level of eighteen-year-old deaf students was at a third-grade level, and the mean mathematics performance was at a sixth- to seventh-grade level. Hearing students' reading and math tests at fifteen years of age (few students over fifteen years old take the Stanford Achievement Test) showed a median performance of a tenth-grade equivalent in both areas (Allen, 1986). It was concluded that hearing-impaired students lag behind their hearing counterparts in reading and mathematics. However, the researcher cautioned that careful descriptions of subgroups of the population, including the region of the country, school program, ethnic group, degree of hearing loss, and additional disabilities, must be taken into account when evaluating students' performance. Through research and program development, professionals in the fields of education, anthropology, sociology, psychology, mental health, and linguistics continue to explore these complex and controversial issues in educational and developmental aspects of deafness (Moores and Meadow-Orlans, 1990).

CULTURE

Deaf persons' cumulative experiences through family and school environments and their social interactions with deaf and hearing peers and adults help shape their cultural perspectives. Some deaf adults are part of the hearing culture; others, although they live and work with hearing people, are members of the Deaf culture. A large number of people who have a progressive hearing loss or who develop hearing loss in adulthood may feel that they are caught between hearing and Deaf cultures, resulting in a great sense of isolation. Communicating with the hearing world becomes difficult or tiresome; speech may no longer be understood without visual clues, and the use of voice telephone is difficult or impossible. These individuals may also feel uncomfortable with culturally Deaf individuals because of beginning signing skills or a lack of common experience.

"A culture is a set of learned behaviors of a group of people who have their own language, values, rules for behavior and traditions" (Padden, 1980). The Deaf population in the United States is a closely knit group bound together by history, language, and common experience. A Deaf person may be born into Deaf culture, as is the case with those who have Deaf parents, or may become enculturated later in life. Since the majority of deaf individuals are from hearing families, the great majority of individuals who are part of the Deaf culture do not join at birth but choose it themselves, in contrast to most cultures (Padden and Humphries, 1988).

An important value of Deaf culture is respect for its language, ASL (Padden, 1980). Through ASL, Deaf people learn about their culture and share experiences (Baker and Cokely, 1980). The exact number of Deaf people in the United States is not known; however, it is estimated that two hundred and fifty thousand to five hundred thousand people in the United States and Canada use ASL (Baker and Cokely, 1980; Padden and Humphries, 1988).

In general, Deaf people disassociate themselves from speech. Among a group of Deaf people, speech is almost never used. That a deaf person does not use speech may be an indication not of that person's ability to use speech but rather of Deaf cultural values. However, some Deaf persons may use speech in situations where they would not otherwise be understood, such as with hearing persons (Padden and Humphries, 1988). The degree of hearing loss does not necessarily determine a person's cultural identity: many Deaf people audiologically have a mild or moderate hearing loss; conversely, individuals with a severe to profound loss are not necessarily Deaf.

Culturally Deaf people see their deafness not as a disability but as a cultural difference. Padden and Humphries (1988) stated that "'disabled' is a label that historically has not belonged to Deaf people. It suggests political self-representations and goals unfamiliar to the group. When Deaf people discuss their deafness, they use terms deeply related to their language, their past, and their community" (p. 44). This view may be reflected by the preference of the Deaf community for the terms *Deaf* (the cultural viewpoint) or *deaf/hard of hearing* (the audiologic viewpoint) rather than *hearing impaired*. Bienvenu (1989) described *hearing impaired* as a derogatory, negative term that does not show respect for the Deaf community. However, other individuals (deaf and hearing), including parents of a child with hearing loss, may prefer to use *hearing impaired,* seeing this as a more polite, less threatening term. Therefore, how individuals refer to themselves (or to a family member) may give important information about their cultural ties and perspective on deafness.

Deaf people tend to socialize within their cultural group. Across the country Deaf people interact in Deaf clubs and organizations, both social and political. Approximately 90 percent of deaf people (culturally Deaf or not) marry another deaf person (Schein, 1989). Additionally, many Deaf persons feel that it would be more desirable to have deaf children because of the communication ties and the strong desire to preserve Deaf culture (Bienvenu and Colonomus, 1985).

COMMUNICATION

Deaf people in the United States use a wide range of communication options, which may include manual communication (sign language), speech / speechreading, and writing / reading. Some deaf individuals may be proficient in only one type of communication; others may use a combination of communication systems, depending on the setting and whether they are communicating with deaf or hearing persons. Telephone communication for the deaf individual may occur through voice with the assistance of hearing aids and telephone amplifiers, through the use of interpreters or relay services, or through assistive devices called telecommunication devices for the deaf.

Sign Language

Sign language is the preferred means of communicating for many deaf individuals. Sign language is a general term that may include a variety of types of manual communication. In the United States, the language used by many Deaf people is American Sign Language. A linguistically recognized language that differs from English, ASL is a visual-gestural language created by Deaf people and has its own history, grammar, syntax, and idioms. The grammar and syntax are expressed through specific movements and shapes of the hands and arms, eyes, face, head, and body posture (Baker and Cokely, 1980; Bellugi, 1980).

ASL differs from other forms of sign communication. A number of systems have been created to represent English manually. Although these systems may borrow from ASL, they use English grammar, syntax, and meaning. Some systems used today include Signing Exact English and Signed

English (National Information Center on Deafness, 1987a). Some users of English sign systems simultaneously use spoken English. Another form of sign communication is Pidgin Signed English (PSE), combining elements of ASL and English that evolved naturally from situations in which users of ASL interacted with users of English (Baker and Cokely, 1980).

Knowledge of and/or proficiency in one type of manual communication does not necessarily indicate that a person can communicate effectively using another type of sign language. ASL structure differs so much from English structure that it would be impossible for a person simultaneously to speak full English sentences and sign the same message in ASL (Johnson, Liddell, and Erting, 1989). Additionally, sign language varies from country to country and may even vary within regions of the same country. Therefore, deaf and hearing people who know one sign language cannot necessarily communicate with other deaf people around the world. However, a separate international sign system (Gestuno) has been developed, which allows deaf and hearing individuals from across the world to communicate with others who know this sign system.

Oral Communication

Some deaf individuals communicate orally, through the use of voice and speechreading (lipreading). Others may use this mode in combination with a signed (English) system, or in situations where they would not otherwise be understood. A deaf person's use of voice or voice quality may not indicate the degree of hearing loss or ability to understand speech. Speech therapy, residual hearing, the use of hearing aids, and the onset of hearing loss after the development of speech may all contribute to a deaf person's use and quality of speech. Profoundly deaf individuals may have very intelligible speech but be unable to hear a conversation, and speechreading skills may vary.

Speechreading is the ability to understand a speaker's spoken communication by watching the movement of the lips, face, and body. Situational clues and prior knowledge of the language being used are important tools. The amount and type of training and the degree of language comprehension contribute to the development of good speechreading skills (Kaplan, Bally, and Garretson, 1987). Speechreading training requires instruction about visually confusing phonemes, which are the smallest unit of speech distinguishing one sound from another (Katz, 1985). For example, many sounds look the same on the lips, and many sounds may be either invisible or difficult to see (Rodel, 1985). However, it is also believed that some individuals have a natural aptitude for speechreading. Kaplan and coworkers (1987) concluded that intelligence, degree and duration of hearing loss, and educational level do not seem to be associated with the level of speechreading skill.

Several factors can interfere with accurate speechreading. If the speaker limits his or her mouth opening or lip movements, this can make it difficult to speechread. However, speech that is exaggerated or slowed for the benefit of the speechreader may distort the visible patterns of speech. Other factors that can interfere with accurate speechreading include mumbling, talking with hands over the mouth, or poor eye contact. A mustache or beard may make speechreading more difficult if the speaker's mouth is partially or totally covered. Additional factors may include settings where the deaf person is likely to experience anxiety, stress, fatigue, unfamiliar terminology, and poor or inadequate lighting (DiPietro, Knight, and Sams, 1981; Kaplan, Bally, and Garretson, 1987). While some deaf individuals may be skilled speechreaders, others are not or may prefer not to rely on this form of communication. Therefore, effective communication through speechreading may depend on a combination of factors, including the skills of the deaf person and the hearing speaker, as well as the situation and setting where the interaction takes place.

Telephone Communication

Some deaf individuals are able to communicate on the telephone through the use of voice, with the assistance of hearing aids and/or telephone amplifiers. However, many people with severe to profound deafness are not able to communicate on the telephone using voice. Telecommunication devices (called TTYs) enable deaf people to type phone messages over the telephone network directly to another person who has this same equipment. A TTY may be portable and resembles a typewriter with an additional device that accommodates the handset of a regular telephone. The conversation is printed on a display area, so that communicators can see the conversation. Some TTYs have the ability to print the entire conversation on paper so that a record can be maintained.

A TTY message-relay system is an alternative for a deaf person who wants to contact someone who does not have a TTY. Through a service operator, a deaf person can indirectly contact a person who uses voice phone, and vice versa. The message is relayed word for word through the operator to the deaf and hearing persons.

The need for genetic counseling for deaf individuals and their families has been recognized for several years (Nance, 1971, 1977). Traditionally, genetic counseling has been utilized by hearing parents of deaf children who may be concerned with the etiology of deafness in their child, medical intervention, and the "risk" of having other deaf children. Nance and coauthors (1977) suggested that counseling may be even more relevant for deaf adults who want to learn about the cause of their deafness and who have questions related to childbearing. Even individuals with known environmental causes of hearing loss can benefit from genetic counseling, providing the first opportunity for the deaf individual to discover how the environmental event actually caused the hearing loss, and how this may affect future children. Deaf people with congenital rubella syndrome may have an increased risk of developing diabetes and thyroid disease (Clarke et al., 1984; Shaver et al., 1984). Genetic counseling that includes information about these risks can be an important part of the overall health care of these individuals. Additionally, the deaf adult, as a member of the general population, may also be at risk for birth defects or genetic conditions based on maternal age, family history, and / or ethnic background, and may seek genetic counseling for information related to these issues.

For the deaf client who may not view deafness as a handicap and who may have a great sense of pride in being Deaf, traditional medical terms used in genetic counseling may create barriers to accessing genetic services and for effective genetic counseling to occur (Arnos, 1990). Terms such as *risk, aVected,* and *abnormal* tend to suggest that deafness is a handicap and may reflect a hearing cultural bias. Culturally Deaf individuals may see geneticists as professionals who want to change or "cure" genes for deafness. Therefore, the Deaf couple who prefer to have deaf children may not be motivated to seek genetic counseling in a setting where their cultural and communication choices are perceived to be misunderstood. The genetic professional's conscious use of neutral words, such as the "chance" to have "hearing" or "deaf" children may contribute to successful communication.

The communication preferences and needs of deaf people can present one of the most significant obstacles to the delivery of health care (Lass et al., 1978; Schein and Delk, 1980; DiPietro, Knight, and Sams, 1981; McEwen and Anton-Culver, 1988). The genetic staff's knowledge of the language and communication issues related to deafness is the first step toward challenging this potential barrier.

In genetic counseling, no single mode of communication will work best for every deaf client. The type of communication used with each deaf client will depend on the deaf person's preferred means of communication, which may be sign language, oral communication, reading and writing, or a combination of these modes.

Legal Issues

In 1973, Section 504 of the Rehabilitation Act was established to protect the deaf person's right to effective communication in health care agencies that receive federal funding. In accordance with this law, each health care agency develops a central office within the agency responsible for coordinating communication services for deaf patients. This office has a full list of available communication options for the agency's deaf patients, which may include qualified sign and oral interpreters, flash cards, supplementary hearing devices, and written communications. More recently, through the enactment of Title III of the Americans with Disabilities Act (ADA), places of public accommodation (including doctors' offices, regardless of the office size or number of employees, hospitals, health clinics, nursing homes, etc.) must provide "auxiliary aids and services" to ensure effective communication with individuals who are deaf or hard of hearing (DuBow, Geer, and Strauss, 1992). If the deaf client requests an interpreter, the agency is responsible for obtaining an interpreter at no additional cost to the client (National Center for Law and the Deaf, 1988, 1989; DuBow, Geer, and Strauss, 1992). Hospital administrators and the U.S. Department of Justice (Civil Rights Division) can assist health care staff in learning how to comply with these laws.

The 504 law mandates TTYs in health care agencies that receive federal funding. Title IV of the ADA of 1990 requires that telecommunication services be expanded to benefit individuals with hearing loss. Currently, telephone companies are required to provide both intra- and interstate telephone relay services. The ADA requires that relay services be available twenty-four hours a day, seven days a week, without any restrictions on the type or length of the call or on the number of calls that can be made by a relay user (DuBow, Geer, and Strauss, 1992).

The availability of telephone communication for deaf individuals— either directly through the use of TTYs within the genetic center or hospital, or indirectly through relay services—can reduce barriers to accessing genetic and medical services. Additionally, these services offer a means for deaf individuals to follow up on questions that may develop and/or to clarify information after a visit.

Using an Interpreter

Interpreters (sign and oral) can offer one of the most effective ways of facilitating communication between hearing and deaf persons (N.J. Department of Human Services, 1990). The role of the interpreter is to convey accurately all messages between deaf and hearing individuals. The interpreter has the obligation to interpret everything that is said, using the communication mode most easily understood or preferred by the deaf person. If the deaf person's preferred mode of communication is an English sign system, the message may be presented word for word. If ASL is used, the interpreter may depart from the exact words, where concepts and idioms are presented in a more descriptive way. The interpreter strives to convey as accurately as possible the speaker's thoughts, feelings, and attitudes, to retain the meaning of the original message. The interpreter does not enter into the conversation, voice personal opinions, or edit the conversation while interpreting (Reisman, Scanlon, and Kemp, 1977; N.J. Department of Human Services, 1990).

The Registry of Interpreters for the Deaf (RID) established a national certification system to test the skills, ethics, and professional behavior of interpreters. There are different levels of certification, depending on the interpreter's skill in ASL and English. Oral interpreters may also be certified (Frishberg, 1986). The 504 law and ADA do not require that interpreters be certified, but they must be qualified. A staff person who "knows sign language" may not necessarily be qualified to interpret adequately. Additionally, problems may arise when a family member or friend acts as an interpreter because of confidentiality and / or emotional issues that may be involved.

Just as there are different levels of interpreter based on their signing skill, there are specialty areas in which an interpreter may or may not be proficient, including legal, mental health, and medical matters. Medical interpreters may be knowledgeable about some of the procedures involved in a genetic counseling appointment, such as the terminology used in taking a family and medical history and the physical exam (Barnum and Siebert, 1987), but may have limited exposure to some of the technical genetic terminology. Contacting and / or meeting the interpreter before the appointment to review the counseling process and genetic terms will help facilitate communication during the session. Some interpreters may find it useful to have a list of words with their meanings before the counseling session.

Working with deaf clients through an interpreter or directly through oral or written modes is a challenge to the counselor's goal of accurate and clear communication. Table 13.1 gives tips that may improve communication either directly or when an interpreter is used. In either situation, it is essential that the counselor assess the deaf client's understanding of the information throughout the session. Nodding by the client, as if indicating understanding, should not be interpreted as comprehension. It may be useful for the counselor to rephrase information if a point is not clear, or to ask the client to summarize what has been discussed to check on his or her understanding of the material. Clear, concise, organized information that is complemented by the use of visual charts or illustrations whenever possible can help describe concepts (Jensen, 1985). Due to the communication needs of deaf clients, modifications can be made in how and when visual charts are used. For example, a hearing client can "listen" to an explanation and focus on an illustration at the same time (and does not need to maintain eye contact with the counselor during this time). This process is different for the deaf client, who is relying on visual cues for communication. In this situation, the counselor must continue to maintain eye contact with the deaf client while giving an explanation, before moving to the illustration. In this way, valuable information will not be missed during the client's transition from one visual medium to another.

Medical and Family History Information

As with all clients, counselors should be aware from the outset of the deaf person's educational background and previous exposure to medical terminology. Some deaf individuals may have had little exposure to medical terms (Schein and Delk, 1980; McEwen and Anton-Culver, 1988) and may never have had a biology or genetics course. Some deaf individuals had limited discussions about health care at home, work, or school, or have had fewer opportunities for incidental learning about the health care process through television and radio. Additionally, printed materials about health care topics that are available to the deaf person may not be written at the appropriate reading level for the average deaf adult. In a study by Lass and coworkers (1978), the words *nausea* and *allergic* were found not to be well understood by a deaf population when presented in written form. Similarly, McEwen and Anton-Culver (1988) noted that fewer than 50 percent of their population could correctly identify the meaning of "gallbladder, stools, sober, anxiety, erection, and nausea." DiPietro and coworkers (1981) reported that some deaf college students have been known to confuse the terms *constipation* and *diarrhea* or believe them to be identical.

Table 13.1. Suggestions for Communicating with Deaf People

1. Face the deaf individual. If using an interpreter, speak directly to the client; do not say "tell him" or "ask her" to the interpreter.

2. Maintain eye contact with the deaf person while speaking.

3. Be aware of your facial expressions and body language when talking.

4. Have adequate lighting, so that the deaf person can see your and / or the interpreter's face without interference of bright light.

5. Speak clearly at a normal pace and volume. If the deaf person does not understand what you have said (directly or through the interpreter), try rephrasing or rewording the sentence.

6. When speaking, do not cover your mouth or have objects such as pens close to your mouth.

7. Have only one person talk at a time.

Source: Data from Kaplan, Bally, and Garretson (1987); New Jersey Department of Human Services (1990)

Some deaf individuals have a limited knowledge of their past medical history. Since the majority (90 percent) of deaf persons come from hearing families, there may have been fewer opportunities for interaction and communication with family members to learn about health care and their own past medical history. Additionally, because of communication barriers between themselves and the medical community, facts about their medical history may not have been fully understood (DiPietro, Knight, and Sams, 1981; DiPietro and Knight, 1982). Therefore, medical history may need to be documented through requests for medical and audiologic records.

Family history information is also limited for some deaf individuals. Knowledge of the family history or access to this information may again result from poor communication at home and should not be considered a reflection of intelligence or lack of desire to learn this information. To help the deaf client obtain this information, forms written at an appropriate reading level with questions about the client's medical and family history can be sent in advance of the appointment with recommendations that the client share this form with his or her family. Additionally, the genetic professional can offer to contact the client's family directly to review this information.

Communication barriers may contribute to a deaf person's lack of knowledge and / or understanding of the health care process. These obstacles may also limit a deaf person's access to genetic services and interfere with successful genetic counseling. However, deaf persons' perception of genetic counseling may also be influenced by their cultural definition of deafness, how they view their own deafness, and their preferences for deaf or hearing children.

CONCLUSION

Deafness is heterogeneous, having many genetic and environmental causes. Genetic types of deafness may be congenital or may develop in childhood or adulthood; the degree of hearing loss may range from mild to profound and can be progressive. Deaf individuals and their families can benefit from genetic services to learn about the etiology of deafness, medical considerations, and childbearing issues. Traditionally, genetic centers across the country mainly serve hearing parents of deaf children, but have seen relatively few deaf adults in genetic counseling who may be seeking information related to the etiology of their deafness and/or unrelated issues. This may be due in part to the cultural, linguistic, and communication differences of this group. When deaf adults do seek genetic services, cultural, linguistic, and communication factors may also create barriers to successful genetic counseling.

Deaf people view their deafness in different ways. Some deaf individuals who are part of the hearing culture see their deafness as a "handicap" and are concerned about the "risk" for future children to be deaf. Other deaf individuals are culturally Deaf and see their deafness not as a "disability" but as a cultural difference. These values may be reflected in a Deaf's person's views on marriage and family; he or she may prefer deaf children and may consider hearing children a "risk." Neutral medical terms that reflect an understanding of Deaf culture, such as *chance, deaf, hearing,* can be used in place of traditional medical terms such as *risk, affected,* and *normal.*

Individuals who are deaf may feel part of the hearing or deaf culture, or may feel that their needs are not met by either group. Several national organizations, including the National Association of the Deaf (NAD), A. G. Bell Association for the Deaf, Self Help for Hard of Hearing People, Inc. (SHHH), and the Association of Late Deafened Adults (ALDA), provide social support and advocacy.

Deaf people are individuals whose cultural beliefs, language, and modes of communication may vary. Some deaf individuals communicate through sign language; others prefer oral communication through speech and speechreading. Communication through writing may complement other modes of communication. However, for some deaf individuals who have poor reading and writing skills, communication solely by written form not only may be time-consuming but also may limit what the deaf person can understand.

In preparing for the deaf client, it is essential that the counselor have a knowledge of the deaf person's preferred mode of communication. The deaf client can be asked in advance whether he or she prefers a sign language interpreter (ASL or English sign language), an oral interpreter, or direct communication. If he or she requests an interpreter, the counselor should contact the administrative office within the hospital or agency to determine who is responsible for coordinating communication services for deaf clients. Health care agencies are required by Section 504 of the 1973 Rehabilitation Act or through Title III of the Americans with Disabilities Act to provide an interpreter at no additional cost to the client. Genetic centers can develop communication guidelines on how to work with deaf clients based on their hospital's or agency's requirements. Local interpreting services and the Registry of Interpreters for the Deaf, Inc., a national organization located in Rockville, Maryland, can provide additional information on the availability of interpreters in specific regions of the country.

Telephone communication devices (TTYs) and relay services may help to increase the utilization of genetic services by deaf people. Genetic counselors spend countless hours on the telephone with clients, making appointments, discussing the genetic counseling process, and gathering information for visits and for follow-up information. TTYs are relatively inexpensive and are portable. A genetic center that serves or expects to serve many deaf individuals may want to purchase a TTY. Agencies that receive federal funding and other health care facilities will have a TTY available for general use by all staff members. An alternative to using a TTY for communication is a relay service. Title IV of the ADA requires telephone companies to provide both local and long-distance telecommunication relay services. The availability of relay services will increase access to genetic centers by deaf individuals.

Lectures and workshops may be provided to deaf groups, parent groups, medical professionals, audiologists, and special-interest groups in deafness. With an awareness of the cultural, linguistic, and communication issues that influence genetic counseling, geneticists and genetic counselors can network with professionals who serve deaf clients, and can educate deaf individuals and their family members about the benefits of genetic counseling services.

SUMMARY

—Do not refer to deafness as a disability or handicap, since some individuals may not view their deafness in this way. (If deafness is not considered a disability by the deaf client, then giving birth to a deaf child will probably not be considered a problem.)

—Ascertain how the patient refers to himself or herself—deaf, hard of hearing, hearing impaired—and refer to the person in the same way.

—Before the counseling session, determine the means of communication: sign language (what type), writing, speechreading. Arrange for a sign language interpreter, if needed. Make sure the patient is comfortable and understands the particular sign language being used.

—Prepare a list of genetic terminology and definitions for the interpreter. If possible, give this to the interpreter before the counseling session so that he or she can be familiar with specific signs.

—Access TTYs for telephone communication (i.e., taking family histories before the counseling session). Local telephone companies provide an operator relay service so that the genetic center does not need to possess a TTY to communicate with someone who has one.

—Do not use the terms *abnormal* or *affected* in referring to deaf individuals. Instead, refer to genes as *altered,* and discuss the *chance* involved.

—The use of visual aids is extremely useful. Be careful not to attempt to communicate while pictures are being viewed.

—Family medical history may need to be documented through medical records or hearing family members. Send family history questionnaires out before any visit.

—Educational levels vary because of resources available to deaf individuals. Determine if the patient has had science education, which would provide a background for understanding some of the terminology and concepts discussed in the counseling session. Adapt the presentation to the patient's educational level.

ACKNOWLEDGMENTS

We thank Robert C. Johnson, Dorothy Smith, and Mitzi Bramble for their editorial assistance.

This work was supported in part by project MCJ–111005–06 from the Maternal and Child Health Program (Title V, Social Security Act), Health Resources and Services Administration, Department of Health and Human Services.

An earlier version of this chapter appeared as "Genetic Counseling for Deaf Adults:

Communication / Language and Cultural Considerations," *Journal of Genetic Counseling* 1
(June 1992):135–53.

REFERENCES

Allen, T. E. 1986. Patterns of academic achievement among hearing impaired students, 1974
and 1983. In Schildroth, A. N., and Karchmer, M. A. (eds.), *Deaf Children in America,*
pp. 161–206. San Diego: College-Hill Press.

Arnos, K. S. 1990. Special considerations in genetic counseling with the Deaf population.
Birth Defects 26:199–202.

Baker, C., and Cokely, D. 1980. *American Sign Language: A Teacher's Resource Text on Grammar and Culture,* pp. 47–60. Silver Spring, Md.: T. J. Publishers.

Barker, D. F., Hostikka, S. L., Zhou, J., Chow, L. T., Oliphant, A. R., Gerken, S. C., Gre-
gory, M. C., Skolnick, M. H., Atkin, C. L., and Tryggvason, K. 1990. Identification of
mutations in the COL45A collagen gene in Alport syndrome. *Science* 248:1224–27.

Barnum, M., and Siebert, E. 1987. *Interpreting in Medical Settings: A Student Manual,* pp.
1–184. St. Paul: St Mary's Campus.

Bellugi, U. 1980. How signs express complex meanings. In Baker, C., and Battison, R.
(eds.), *Sign Language and the Deaf Community: Essays in Honor of William C. Stokoe,* pp.
53–74. Silver Spring, Md.: National Association of the Deaf.

Bergstrom, L. V. 1980. Causes of severe hearing loss in early childhood. *Pediatric Annals*
9:22–30.

Bienvenu, M. J. 1989. An open letter to alumni, students of Gallaudet, and friends. *Bicul-
tural Center News* 18:1–8.

Bienvenu, M. J., and Colonomus, B. 1985. *An Introduction to American Deaf Culture,* Part
2: Values. Videocassette. Silver Spring, Md.: Sign Media.

Biesecker, B., Magyari, P. A., and Paul, N. W. (eds). 1987. Strategies in genetic counseling.
II: Religious, cultural, and ethnic influences on the counseling process. *Birth Defects*
23:1–281.

Boughman, J. A., and Shaver, K. A. 1982. Genetic aspects of deafness: Understanding the
counseling process. *American Annals of the Deaf* 127:393–400.

Clarke, W. L., Shaver, K. A., Bright, G. M., Rogol, A. D., and Nance, W. E. 1984. Autoim-
munity in congenital rubella syndrome. *Journal of Pediatrics* 104:370–73.

Davenport, S. L. H. 1977. Improving communication with the deaf patient. *Journal of Family Practice* 4:1065–68.

DiPietro, L. J., and Knight, C. H. 1982. When your patient is deaf. *Professional Medical
Assistant* 15:16–23.

DiPietro, L. J., Knight, C. H., and Sams, J. S. 1981. Health care delivery for deaf patients:
The provider's role. *American Annals of the Deaf* 126:106–12.

DuBow, S., Geer, S., and Strauss, K. P. 1992. *Legal Rights: The Guide for Deaf and Hard of
Hearing People: Featuring the Americans with Disabilities Act!* 4th ed., pp. 15–45. Washington, D.C.: Gallaudet University Press.

Foy, C., Newton, V., Wellesley, D., Harris, R., and Read, A. P. 1990. Assignment of the locus for Waardenburg syndrome type I to human chromosome 2q37 and possible homology to the splotch mouse. *American Journal of Human Genetics* 46:1017–23.

Fraser, G. R. 1976. *The Causes of Profound Deafness in Childhood.* Baltimore: Johns Hopkins University Press.

Frishberg, N. 1986. *Interpreting: An Introduction,* pp. 87–145. Rockville, Md.: RID Publications.

Gorlin, R. J., Toriello, H. V., and Cohen, M. M. 1995. *Hereditary Hearing Loss and Its Syndromes.* New York: Oxford University Press.

Hotchkiss, D. 1989. *Demographic Aspects of Hearing Impairment: Questions and Answers.* 2d ed. Gallaudet Research Institute. Washington, D.C.: Gallaudet University.

Israel, J. 1989. Counseling in Deaf/hearing impaired adult populations. *Perspectives in Genetic Counseling* 11:1, 4.

Jensen, K. M. 1985. Communicating of the diagnosis to the deaf family. *Birth Defects* 21:69–84.

Johnson, R. E., Liddell, S. K., and Erting, C. J. 1989. Unlocking the curriculum: Principles for achieving access in deaf education. Gallaudet Research Institute Working Paper 89–3, pp. 1–29. Washington, D.C.: Gallaudet University.

Kaplan, H., Bally, S. J., and Garretson, C. 1987. *Speechreading: A Way to Improve Understanding.* 2d ed., pp. 1–17. Washington, D.C.: Gallaudet University Press.

Katz, J. (ed.). 1985. *Handbook of Clinical Audiology.* 3d ed., p. 1082. Baltimore: Williams and Wilkins.

Kimberling, W. J., Weston, M. D., Moller, C., van Aaren, A., Cremers, C. W. R. J., Sumegi, J., Ing, P., Connolly, C., Martini, A., Milani, M., Tamayo, M. L., Bernal, J., Greenberg, J., Ayuso, C. 1995. Gene mapping of Usher syndrome type IIA: Localization of the gene to a 2.1–cM segment on chromosome 1q41. *American Journal of Human Genetics* 56:216–23.

Konigsmark, B. W., and Gorlin, R. J. 1976. *Genetic and Metabolic Deafness.* Philadelphia: W. B. Saunders.

Kumar, S., Kimberling, W. J., Connolly, C. J., Tinley, S., Marres, H. A. M., and Cremers, C. W. R. J. 1994. Refining the region of branchio-oto-renal syndrome and defining the flanking markers on chromosome 8q by genetic mapping. *American Journal of Human Genetics* 55:1188–94.

Langham-Brown, S. J. 1981. Problems of communication in patient care. *Nursing Times* (11 June):1035–37.

Lass, L. G., Franklin, R. R., Bertrand, W. E., and Baker, J. 1978. Health knowledge, attitudes, and practices of the deaf population in the greater New Orleans: A pilot study. *American Annals of the Deaf* 123:960–67.

Lewis, R. A., Otterud, B., Stauffer, D., Lalouel, J. M., and Leppert, M. 1990. Mapping recessive ophthalmic diseases: Linkage of the locus for Usher syndrome type II to a DNA marker on chromosome 1q. *Genomics* 7:250–56.

McEwen, E., and Anton-Culver, H. 1988. The medical communication of deaf patients. *Journal of Family Practice* 26:289–91.

Meadow-Orlans, K. P. 1990. Research on developmental aspects of deafness. In Moores,

D. F., and Meadow-Orlans, K. P. (eds.), *Educational and Developmental Aspects of Deafness*, pp. 283–98. Washington, D.C.: Gallaudet University Press.

Meyers, J. E., Melhado, J. J., and Frances, D. R. 1989. Hearing impaired patients in the medical setting. *Journal of the American Osteopathic Association* 89:780–82.

Moores, D. F. 1990. Research in educational aspects of deafness. In Moores, D. F., and Meadow-Orlans, K. P. (eds.), *Educational and Developmental Aspects of Deafness*, pp. 11–24. Washington, D.C.: Gallaudet University Press.

Moores, D. F., and Meadow-Orlans, K. P. (eds.). 1990. *Educational and Developmental Aspects of Deafness*, pp. 1–451. Washington, D.C.: Gallaudet University Press.

Nance, W. E. 1971. Genetic counseling for the hearing impaired. *Audiology* 10:222–33.

———. 1977. Genetic counseling of hereditary deafness: An unmet need. In Bess, F. H. (ed.), *Childhood Deafness: Causation, Assessment, and Management*, pp. 211–16. New York: Grune and Stratton.

Nance, W. E., Rose, S. P., Conneally, P. M., and Miller, J. Z. 1977. Opportunities for genetic counseling through institutional ascertainment of affected probands. In Lubs, H. A., and de la Cruz, F. F. (eds.), *Genetic Counseling*, pp. 307–31. New York: Raven Press.

National Center for Law and the Deaf. 1988. *Guidelines for Hospital Policy for Hearing-Impaired Patients*. Washington, D.C.: Gallaudet University.

———. 1989. *Section 504: A Law to Stop Discrimination against Disabled Persons*, pp. 1–9. Washington, D.C.: Gallaudet University.

National Information Center on Deafness. 1987a. *Deafness: A Fact Sheet*. Washington, D.C.: Gallaudet University.

———. 1987b. *Educating Deaf Children: An Introduction*. Washington, D.C.: Gallaudet University.

New Jersey Department of Human Services, Division of Deaf and Hard of Hearing. 1990. *Deafness and Interpreting*. Trenton: New Jersey Department of Human Services.

Padden, C. A. 1980. The deaf community and culture of deaf people. In Baker, C., and Battison, R. (eds.), *Sign Language and the Deaf Community: Essays in Honor of William C. Stokoe*, pp. 89–103. Silver Spring, Md.: National Association of the Deaf.

Padden, C. A., and Humphries, T. L. 1988. *Deaf in America: Voices from a Culture*. Cambridge: Harvard University Press.

Paul, N., and Kavanagh, L. (eds.). 1990. National symposium on genetic services for underserved populations. *Birth Defects* 26:1–290.

Rawlings, B. W., and Jensema, C. J. 1977. Two studies of the families of hearing impaired children. Gallaudet University, Office of Demographic Studies, ser. R, no. 5. Washington, D.C.: Gallaudet University.

Reisman, G., Scanlan, J., and Kemp, K. 1977. Medical interpreting for hearing impaired patients. *Journal of the American Medical Association* 237:2397–98.

Rodel, M. J. 1985. Children with hearing impairment. In Katz, J. (ed.), *Handbook of Clinical Audiology*. 3d ed., pp. 1004–16. Baltimore: Williams and Wilkins.

Rose, S. P., Conneally, P. M., and Nance, W. E. 1977. Genetic analysis of childhood deafness. In Bess, F. H. (ed.), *Childhood Deafness*, pp. 19–35. New York: Grune and Stratton.

Schein, J. D. 1989. *At Home among Strangers,* pp. 106–34. Washington, D.C.: Gallaudet University Press.

Schein, J. D., and Delk, M. T. 1980. Survey of health care for deaf people. *Deaf American* 32:5, 6, 27.

Shaver, K. A., Boughman, J. A., Kenyon, N., Mohanakumar, T., and Nance, W. E. 1984. HLA antigens in the congenital rubella syndrome. *Disease Markers* 2:381–91.

Wood, T. E. 1987. Communicating with hearing impaired patients. *Journal of the American Optometric Association* 58:62–65.

Index

Birth control: Amish and, 179; Asian Indians and, 145, 147; Koreans and, 139; Latinos and, 23; Native Americans and, 79; Roman Catholicism and, 23, 158–59, 173; Southeast Asians and, 124

Birth defects, 13–14, 77, 93, 125, 134, 139

Birth rates: Amish, 177; Hispanic, 22

Blood loss, 120, 123–24

Blood transfusions, 163

Borrego, R. L., 26

Bosque Redondo, Treaty of (1868), 63

Bowman, J. E., 45–46

Buddhism: in China, 89; in Japan, 101, 102; in Korea, 130, 131, 139; in Southeast Asia, 114, 115

California, 21, 99

Calvin, John, 161

Cambodians, 113, 114, 116, 118, 120, 123, 124

Canada, 99, 100, 153

Cancer, 31–32, 109

Carlton, James, 63

Carson, Kit, 63

Caudill, W., 8

Chamberlain, N., 41

Chavez, E. L., 26

Chesney, A. P., 28

Chiang Kai-shek, 88

Childbirth, 46, 186–87, 212–13

Children: African Americans and, 52; Amish and, 180–81, 193; Asian Indians and, 152; Chinese and, 90; Christians and, 165, 170; deafness and, 221–22, 233; European Americans and, 4–5, 7–8, 10, 13; Japanese and, 103–4, 107, 109, 110; Jews and, 209, 213–15; Koreans and, 133; Latinos and, 24–25, 30–31; Native Americans and, 65, 66, 70; Southeast Asians and, 115–16, 121

China, xx, 86, 89, 90

Chinese culture, 86, 96–97; and communication, 88, 91, 92–93; and family, 89–91, 94; and genetic services, 92–95; and health beliefs, 91–92; history of, 2, 86–89; and languages, 88, 92–93; and religion, 89

Chondogyo religion, 132

Chorionic villus sampling, xvii, 79

Christianity, 156, 173–74; in American culture, 3; denominations of, 157–63; and genetic services, 171–73; and health beliefs, 171; history of, 156–57; in Japan, 101; religious beliefs, 163–68; religious practices, 168–71; in Southeast Asia, 121

Chromosome abnormalities, 139

Church of Christ, Scientist, 163

Church of Jesus Christ of Latter Day Saints (Mormons), 162–63

Circumcision, 213

Cleft lip, 26

Columbus, Christopher, 20

Comanche Indians, 72

Communication, xviii–xx; African Americans and, 52–54; Amish and, 183; Chinese and, 88, 91, 92–93; deafness and, 225–27, 228–29, 232, 233–34; European Americans and, 5–6, 11; Japanese and, 104, 108; Koreans and, 132–33; Latinos and, 25–26; Native Americans and, 78, 79; Southeast Asians and, 116–18

Confucianism, 89, 114, 130, 131–32, 139

Confucius, 131, 134

Congregationalists, 162

Consanguinity: African Americans and, 52; Amish and, 190, 191; Chinese and, 95; Christians and, 159; European Americans and, 4–5; Japanese and, 109; Koreans and, 133–34, 137; Latinos and, 30; Native Americans and, 78–79; Southeast Asians and, 119, 123

Consent forms, 138, 189

Conservative Judaism, 207, 214

Constantine I (emperor of Rome), 157

Contraception. See Birth control

Coronado, Francisco Vásquez de, 61

Cortés, Hernan, 20

Cross, H. E., 177

Cuba, 21

Cuban Americans, 21

Cultural diversity, xviii, xx–xxi, 54

Cultural relativism, xiv

Cultural Status Exam, 43–44, 45

Culture, xiv; genetics and, xvi–xvii; race and, xvii–xviii

Curanderismo, 26

Curanderos, 27–28, 29

Cystic fibrosis, xvii, 188

Deafness, 220–21, 233–35; and communication, 225–27, 228–29, 232, 233–34; culture of, 223–25; and genetic services, 228–33; language acquisition and, 221–23

Death: African Americans and, 37; Amish and, 183–84, 186; Asian Indians and, 145, 146, 151; Buddhism and, 102; Christians and, 167–68, 173; European Americans and, 14–15; Hinduism and, 145, 151; Islam and, 146, 151; Japanese and, 102, 109, 110; Jews and, 209–10, 215–17; Koreans and, 138; Latinos and, 24, 31; Native Americans and, 69, 73–74

Dennis, R. E., 38

Dermabrasion, 120

DiPietro, L. J., 231

Disabilities: Christians and, 164, 165; Deaf culture and, 233; European Americans and, 14; Japanese and, 107, 110; Koreans and, 137;

Southeast Asians, 113, 126–27; and communication, 116–18; cultures of, 118–19; and family, 115–16; and genetic services, 122–26; and health beliefs, 119–22; history and migration of, 113–14; and religion, 114–15
Spain, 19, 20, 61–63, 205
Spanish language, 5, 25
Speechreading, 226–27
Suicide, 105, 107, 217
Supernatural illness, 26, 68–69, 119–20
Superstitiousness, 3–4, 92, 105, 152
Surgery, 105, 119–20, 150
Suttee, 149
Swarzentruber Amish, 177

Taegyo, 136
Taoism, 89, 114
Tay Sachs disease, 211
Technology, 10–11, 13, 15. *See also* Reproductive technologies
Telephone communication, deafness and, 227, 229, 234
Texas, 21
Thalassemias, 95, 126
Thomas, R. J., 132
Titley, R. W., 26
Tocqueville, Alexis de, 9
Tokugawa Ieyasu, 99
Toyotomi Hideyoshi, 99, 130

U.S. Census Bureau, 19, 20, 21
U.S. Constitution, 3, 40
U.S. Department of Health and Welfare, 20
U.S. Department of Justice, 229

U.S. Immigration and Naturalization Service, 143
Ultra-Orthodox Jews, 206–7, 210

Vichinsky, E. P., 45
Vietnamese, 113–14, 115–16, 118, 122, 123
Vietnam War, 113, 114
Voodooism, 38

Waltman, G. H., 183, 184, 187
Wang Kon, 130
Western medicine, xv, xviii; African Americans and, 43, 44, 45; Amish and, 178–79, 185; Asian Indians and, 150; Chinese and, 91–92; European Americans and, 15; Japanese and, 106; Koreans and, 136–37; Latinos and, 29; Native Americans and, 73, 80; Southeast Asians and, 122
Williams, D. H., 41
Witchcraft, 26, 50–51, 75–76
Women: African American, 51–52; Asian Indian, 148, 152; Chinese, 90; Japanese, 102–3, 106; Jewish, 206, 208; Korean, 134–35, 136; Muslim, 146, 147; Native American, 64, 65, 67, 69, 75; Southeast Asian, 122
World War II, 87–88, 100

Yiddish language, 205
Yin-yang theory, 92, 105, 119
Yi Songgye, 130
Yupik Eskimos, 80

Zuni Indians, 60, 62, 67

Library of Congress Cataloging-in-Publication Data

Cultural and ethnic diversity : a guide for genetics professionals /
    edited by Nancy L. Fisher.
        p.   cm.
    Includes index.
    ISBN 0-8018-5346-X (hc)
    1. Genetic counseling—United States.   2. Cross-cultural
counseling—United States.   I. Fisher, Nancy L.
RB155.7.C85   1996
616'.042—dc20   96-13763